Manual of Nursing Home Practice for Psychiatrists

The American Psychiatric Association Council on Aging Committee on Long-Term Care and Treatment of the Elderly

James A. Greene, M.D., *Editor and Chair*
Pierre Loebel, M.D., *Co-Editor*
Deborah A. Banazak, D.O.
Joan K. Barber, M.D.
George Dyck, M.D.
Beverly N. Jones, M.D.
Gabe J. Maletta, Ph.D., M.D.
Arturo G. Quiason, M.D.
Elliott M. Stein, M.D.

Contributors

Lory Bright-Long, M.D.
Diane R. Burkett, C.M.M.
Christopher C. Colenda, M.D.
Barry S. Fogel, M.D., M.B.A.
Alan M. Jonas, M.D.
Woody Johnson, L.C.S.W.
Sharon S. Levine, M.D., M.P.H.
Joseph E. V. Rubin, M.D.
Ronald Alan Shellow, M.D.
Joan W. Wagner, R.N., M.S.N.

Reviewers

Daniel B. Borenstein, M.D.
Marion Z. Goldstein, M.D.
George T. Grossberg, M.D.
Samuel W. Kidder, Pharm.D., M.P.H.
Barry W. Rovner, M.D.
Anthony F. Villamena, M.D.

Manual of Nursing Home Practice for Psychiatrists

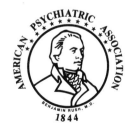

Published by the American Psychiatric Association
Washington, DC

Note: The authors have worked to ensure that all information in this book concerning drug dosages, schedules, and routes of administration is accurate as of the time of publication and consistent with standards set by the U.S. Food and Drug Administration and the general medical community. As medical research and practice advance, however, therapeutic standards may change. For this reason and because human and mechanical errors sometimes occur, we recommend that readers follow the advice of a physician who is directly involved in their care or the care of a member of their family.

The findings, opinions, and conclusions of this report do not necessarily represent the views of the officers, trustees, or all members of the American Psychiatric Association. The views expressed are those of the authors of the individual chapters.

American Psychiatric Association
1400 K Street, N.W., Washington, DC   20005
www.psych.org

Library of Congress Cataloging-in-Publication Data
Manual of nursing home practice for psychiatrists.—1st ed.
    p.   cm.
   Includes bibliographical references and index.
   ISBN 0-89042-283-4 (alk. paper)
   1. Nursing home patients—Mental health services. 2. Mentally ill aged—Nursing home
care. 3. Geriatric psychiatry—Practice—United States.   I. American Psychiatric
Association.
    [DNLM: 1. Mental Health Services. 2. Nursing Homes. 3. Homes for the Aged. 4.
Professional Practice. 5. Psychiatry. WM 30.5 M294 2000]
RC451.4.N87 M36 2000
618.97′689—dc21
                                                                99-048771

British Library Cataloguing in Publication Data
A CIP record is available from the British Library.

Contents

Section 1
Clinical Considerations

Section 2
Regulatory Aspects
OBRA, the Minimum Data Set, and
Other Regulations That Affect Nursing Home Practice

Section 3
Financial Aspects

Section 4
Legal and Ethical Issues

Section 5
Perspectives for the Future

Appendixes

Notice

Medicine is an ever-changing science. As new research and clinical experience broaden our knowledge, changes in treatment and drug therapy are required. The authors and publisher of this work have checked with sources believed to be reliable in their efforts to provide information that is complete and generally in accord with the standards accepted at the time of publication. However, in view of the possibility of human error or changes in medical sciences, neither the authors nor other parties who have been involved in the preparation or publication of this work warrant that the information contained herein is in every respect accurate or complete. They are not responsible for any errors or omissions or for the results obtained from the use of such information. In particular, readers are advised to check the product information sheet included in the package of each drug they plan to administer to be certain the information contained in this book is accurate and that changes have not been made in the recommended dose or in the contraindications for administration. This recommendation is of particular importance in connection with new or infrequently used drugs.

Readers are encouraged to confirm the information contained herein with other sources and update their knowledge about economic mandates and reimbursement. The Health Care Financing Administration, the Health and Human Services Inspector General, and Medicare carriers all are subjecting mental illness treatment claims to intensified scrutiny; thus additional care in documentation is warranted. Consult with your local Medicare carrier, state Medicaid program, and other state and federal regulations regarding changing regulations and regional interpretations.

Foreword

The American Psychiatric Association (APA) Council on Aging has had a distinguished track record in shaping mental health policies and clinical practices for geriatric patients with mental disorders who reside in long-term care settings. In December 1983, the APA Board of Trustees established the Task Force on Nursing Homes and the Mentally Ill. The Task Force was chaired by Dr. Benjamin Liptzin, who was ably assisted by Drs. Soo Borson, James Nininger, and Peter Rabins. They diligently summarized the literature, research findings, and treatment options for mentally ill patients in nursing home settings and made recommendations for future activities in the areas of research, training, and policy. Their work led to the Task Force Report No. 28, *Nursing Homes and the Mentally Ill: A Report of the Task Force of Nursing Homes and Mentally Ill Elderly* (1989) of the American Psychiatric Association. This report followed on the heels of major legislative changes affecting nursing homes as part of the 1987 Omnibus Budget Reconciliation Act, Public Law 100-203 (OBRA-87). The OBRA-87 legislation resulted in large part from a 1986 Institute of Medicine (IOM) of the National Academy of Sciences published report, *Improving the Quality of Care in Nursing Homes.*

From the APA Task Force arose the Committee on Long-Term Care and Treatment of the Elderly. The Committee has been chaired by a number of distinguished psychiatrists, including Drs. Ira Katz, Don Hay, Barry Fogel, and James Greene. The Committee's mission and vision has been focused on improving the quality of care of patients in nursing home settings. To achieve this goal, the Committee has networked successfully with other professional and advocacy groups, including the American Association for Geriatric Psychiatry, the American Geriatrics Society, the American Medical Directors Association, the American Society of Consultant Pharmacists, the American Association for Retired Persons, and the Coalition for Nursing Home Reform.

The years since the 1989 Task Force Report have seen improvements in the quality of care delivered to patients residing in nursing homes. For example, there has been a marked reduction in the use of physical restraints. But the need for high-quality, cost-effective psychiatric services in nursing homes has not lessened over the years. In fact, epidemiologic studies over the past decade have consistently shown that a very high prevalence of psychiatric disorders exists among nursing facility residents. Approximately two of every three residents have diagnosable mental disorders, and one in four has clinically significant symptoms of depression. Further, two-thirds of nursing home residents have dementing illnesses, of which 80% is Alzheimer's disease. The impact of not treating these mental disorders is clear. Untreated, these illnesses lead to increased mortality, further functional disability, worsening symptoms of associated illnesses, and diminished quality of life for vulnerable individuals requiring long-term care services.

In March 1998, the IOM formed the Committee on Improving Quality in Long-Term Care to examine the impact of OBRA-87 legislation on nursing home services. The APA and the American Association for Geriatric Psychiatry provided written testimony to the Committee. The written testimony also recommended strategies to ensure that the delivery of quality mental health services in nursing facilities will be a top priority for any future legislation dealing with long-term care. A key recommendation to the IOM Committee was the development of mental health quality indicators for nursing home residents that make explicit the need for nursing home residents to have access to more affordable, high-quality psychiatric care.

The *Manual of Nursing Home Practice for Psychiatrists* is a timely reference for general psychiatrists, primary care.physicians, and others interested in nursing home practice. It is designed to assist general psychiatrists in understanding the clinical, regulatory, financial, and legal questions associated with nursing home practice. By giving general psychiatrists and other interested professionals this tool, we hope to encourage them to ex-pand their work into nursing facilities and thereby benefit patients who may require psychiatric services.

On behalf of the APA Council on Aging, we thank Drs. James Greene, J. Pierre Loebel, George Dyck, Barry Fogel, Elliott Stein, Joan Barber, Gabe Maletta, Lory Bright-Long, Deb Banazak, and others for their leadership and commitment to producing the *Manual of Nursing Home Practice for Psychiatrists*.

Christopher C. Colenda, M.D., M.P.H.
Chair, Council on Aging
American Psychiatric Association
Professor and Chair
Department of Psychiatry
Michigan State University

Preface

The *Manual of Nursing Home Practice for Psychiatrists* is a product of the American Psychiatric Association Council on Aging and the Committee on Long-Term Care and Treatment of the Elderly.

Its purpose is to give general psychiatrists, primary care physicians, and others with little if any nursing home experience a practical, accurate, and easily readable guide to serve their needs when responding to a consultation request, attending a patient, or exploring the opportunity to accept a position in a skilled nursing home or other long-term care setting.

For ease of reference we have organized the Manual into five sections:

1. Clinical Considerations—information of immediate relevance to patient consultation and the nursing home environment

2. Regulatory Aspects—information regarding OBRA, the Minimum Data Set, and other regulations that have a direct bearing on nursing home practice

3. Financial Aspects—information on how to get paid for services

4. Legal and Ethical Issues

5. Perspectives for the Future

In addition, the appendixes contain a guide to nursing home staffing, sample form letters, useful assessment instruments, and a bibliography to which you may refer for more detailed information.

The Committee also hopes that this manual will stimulate the reader's interest in the rapidly growing field of geriatric psychiatry.

Section 1

Clinical Considerations

Chapter 1

Nursing Homes, Mental Illness, and the Role of the Psychiatrist

Historical Background

The modern nursing home is a unique and remarkable hybrid. It has historical roots whose intertwining and growth have formed our current system of long-term care. These roots have biomedical origins in the acute care hospitals, psychological origins arising from the long-stay mental hospitals (i.e., "asylums"), and social origins in the poorhouse movement of the eighteenth and early nineteenth centuries. Management was at first based on custodial social models. Later the forces contributing to the evolution of nursing homes based their interventions on the medical model. Currently nursing homes are attempting to address the social, psychological, and medical problems that affect their residents. Systems are evolving rapidly that include psychiatric interventions designed to address these complex needs.

As recently as the mid-1970s, aging was viewed as a disease for which there was no intervention except institutionalization or stoic family resolve. Most primary care physicians did not believe that dementia patients could be helped. Many patients were "warehoused" without psychiatric help of any type because they were diagnosed as "senile" or with "hardening of the arteries" and were considered "not treatable." Especially before the development of neuroleptics, antidepressants, and newer anxiolytics, patients were often sedated with phenobarbital or other sedatives. Rarely,

when the patient was extremely psychotic or agitated, a psychiatrist would be consulted.

Psychiatric consultation to nursing homes has been very slow to develop because of inadequate techniques for making the necessary multisystem assessments, ineffective behavioral management of psychiatric symptomatology, and lack of psychiatrist availability and motivation. In addition, psychiatrists have traditionally had little involvement in prescribing psychotropic drugs for long-term residents of nursing homes (Larson and Lyons 1994). More often psychiatric problems have been diagnosed and medications prescribed by primary care physicians.

The burden of behavioral management, therefore, has too frequently fallen onto poorly trained staff who lack the understanding and skills necessary to handle psychopathologic states and their associated behaviors. Overutilization of physical and chemical restraints led to legislative interventions (e.g., the Omnibus Reconciliation Act of 1987 [OBRA-87]) (Rovner and Katz 1994; see also Chapter 5). The "nothing can be done" attitude fulfilled itself as a prophecy and has frequently led to nothing being done (Greene et al. 1985). Clearly with the mushrooming growth of the older population in this country, and advances in psychiatric diagnosis and treatment, this nihilistic attitude must change. We, as psychiatrists with so much to offer older people, must lead the way.

The common public and media belief is that boredom, lack of dignity, a slide into anonymity, over-regimentation, neglect of personal needs, and helplessness will follow admission to the nursing home. Some individuals have committed suicide in response to fear of nursing home placement (Loebel et al. 1991). The psychiatrist who is experienced in this environment will know that in the majority of cases the stereotypes are far from the truth and that the more common milieu is a very supportive and active one, in which the entire biopsychosocial spectrum of patient care receives vigorous attention.

The number of persons served within this system has increased substantially and rapidly. It has been estimated that by the middle of the twenty-first century, more than 1 in every 100 persons in the United States will reside in a nursing home for at least some time. Paralleling these increases and changes in utilization has been a rise in expenditures; various cost-cutting initiatives are now being proposed.

Prevalence of Mental Illness

An extensive epidemiologic literature is now available for the general psychiatrist who is considering nursing home consultation and who may be concerned about the prevalence and severity of the psychiatric disorders that he or she will encounter.

Rovner et al. (1990) estimated rates of schizophrenia at 2.4%, depression at 12.8%, and dementia at 67.4%. The features associated with dementia (e.g., behavioral dyscontrol, depression, delirium, anxiety, psychosis) lead to a request for psychiatric consultation more often than do the cardinal cognitive characteristics of the disorder. Another investigation revealed a moderate to marked degree of cognitive impairment, the presence of mild depression, and moderate to marked levels of overall psychiatric impairment across the entire population studied. According to Borson et al. (1997, p. 1178), "Despite the growth of community care as an alternative to nursing home placement, these results confirm observations made four decades ago and recently renewed that nursing homes care for patients difficult to distinguish

from those treated in acute psychiatric hospitals, emphasizing the need for a full spectrum of mental health services in this setting."

The Role of the Psychiatrist in the Nursing Home

We may conclude that there is a high prevalence of psychopathology among nursing home residents and that this psychopathology manifests itself in symptoms and behaviors that are distressing to patients and that are problematic for their caregivers to manage, many of whom are undertrained and inexperienced. At the same time, lower-grade but pervasively debilitating dysfunctions are often neglected. This situation presents the psychiatrist with an unrivaled scope of practice, of which the ultimate goals are "the maintenance of functional capacity, delaying the progress of disease where possible, and [the] creation of a safe, supportive environment that promotes maximal autonomy and life satisfaction" (Borson et al. 1987, p. 1412).

In addressing these tasks, the roles or functions for which the psychiatrist may be called upon include the following:

- Making accurate diagnoses of complex psychiatric disorders
- Assessing medical, psychological, and social factors that affect patients' functioning
- Applying specialized knowledge and skills in the use of psychoactive medications in this age group, including their efficacy, adverse effects, and interaction with other medications that the patient is likely to be taking
- Documenting assessment and treatment recommendations clearly and concisely, with the needs and nature of the referring staff and physician in mind at all times
- Providing comprehensive and integrated treatment planning, working with the primary care physician and other members of the multidisciplinary staff
- Being proficient in the use of the correct diag-

nostic and billing codes and the proper documentation thereof, in line with Medicare and Medicaid rules and regulations

Aside from diagnosing and treating psychiatric disorders among the individual patients in long-term care facilities, the role of the psychiatrist in the nursing home should include educating and supporting families, primary care physicians, and staff. The scope of this function may include the following activities:

- Encouraging new and appropriate referrals
- Helping staff recognize mental disorders and perceive the patient's symptoms in the context of a medical disorder rather than as willful misconduct, personality traits, or a lack of cooperation
- Reducing problems that cause emotional or behavioral problems in patients through better preventative measures
- Reducing the transmission of myths about mental illness, aging, psychiatric medications, and other psychiatric treatments
- Providing in-service training to nursing staff, physicians, and administration
- Assisting in ensuring compliance with federal and state regulations governing the medical care provided in the particular setting

References

Borson S, Liptzin B, Nininger J, et al: Psychiatry in the nursing home. Am J Psychiatry 144:1412–1418, 1987

Borson S, Loebel JP, Kitchell M, et al: Psychiatric assessments of nursing home residents under OBRA-87: should PASSAR be reformed? J Am Geriatr Soc 45:1173–1181, 1997

Greene JA, Asp J, Crane N: Specialized management of the Alzheimer's disease patient: does it make a difference? a preliminary progress report. J Tenn Med Assoc 78:559–563, 1985

Larson D, Lyons J: The psychiatrist in the nursing home, in The Practice of Psychogeriatric Medicine. New York, Wiley, 1994, p 954

Loebel JP, Loebel JS, Dager SR, et al: Anticipation of nursing home placement may be a precipitant of suicide among the elderly. J Am Geriatr Soc 39:407–408, 1991

Rovner BW, Katz IR: Neuropsychiatry in nursing homes, in The American Psychiatric Press Textbook of Geriatric Neuropsychiatry. Edited by Coffey CE, Cummings JL. Washington, DC, American Psychiatric Press, 1994, p 686

Rovner BW, German PS, Broadhead J, et al: The prevalence and management of dementia and other psychiatric disorders in nursing homes. Int Psychogeriatr 2:13–24, 1990

Chapter 2

Evaluation and Management of Psychiatric Problems in Long-Term Care Patients

The request from a long-term care facility to have a psychiatrist evaluate a patient is an invitation that can lead to a challenging but rewarding relationship, not only with the patient but also with a number of other parties who are already involved with that patient, namely the primary care physician, the patient's family, and the nursing home staff and administration. The nursing home environment is very different from that encountered in the hospital, the institution with which the psychiatrist is likely to be most familiar. Learning the customs and rules of the long-term care facility may take some time and effort, but it can be undertaken as the psychiatrist proceeds carefully and deliberately in examining the patient.

The patient's signs and symptoms should be the psychiatrist's primary concern, but the underlying reasons for the consultation request must be researched carefully. In searching for the etiology of the observed signs of psychiatric illness, the psychiatrist should cast a wide net. Because the nursing home resident is by necessity a person somewhat dependent on his or her environment, the persons who interact with and control that environment take on special importance and cannot be ignored. The time spent in investigating these matters may sometimes seem prohibitive, but the psychiatrist must be forewarned that thoroughness bears a direct relationship to a satisfactory outcome. Like it or not, there will be many persons who either will or will not "sign off" on the treatment plan devised for the patient before it is

implemented fully and completed successfully.

Behavioral symptoms are the most common reason for a psychiatric consultation. These problems often have no clearly discernible cause and are resistant to decisive, quick solutions. Although the psychiatrist is no stranger to complex clinical problems, the nursing home is a special environment that itself needs to be understood in order to manage the patient's problem most effectively within that context. Furthermore, the nursing home staff, the patient, and the family may need help in understanding what the psychiatrist has to offer.

Various factors may lead to a psychiatric consultation, and the psychiatrist must ascertain the reasons behind the request. Because of the stigma attached to psychiatry, some issues may have been disguised or obscured altogether, especially if the psychiatrist is new to a particular setting. Table 2–1 presents a classification of the various reasons that may underlie the consultation request.

Preparation for the Consultation

The psychiatrist needs to be aware that the primary care physician is ultimately in charge of the patient's medical care. The roles of the primary care physician, the nursing home staff, the family, and the patient in initiating the consultation have important implications for how the request is handled.

Table 2–1. Common reasons for psychiatric referral

Patient-centered reasons

Psychiatric illness—threshold is lowest for symptoms that fall outside the usual experience of nursing home staff and attending physicians

Behavioral disturbances (apart from the recognition of psychiatric illness)—may be the most common reason for a referral in some facilities

Illness or death of a spouse, other relative, or friend in or outside the nursing home—not as common as other reasons in this category

Staff-centered reasons

Recognition of a psychiatric problem in the patient

Prejudices and other biases among staff members about norms of conduct

Staff workload and fatigue

Psychiatric referral used as punishment or threat of punishment

Specific behavioral problem on the part of a staff member

Family-centered reasons

Feelings of guilt and uncertainty, especially over nursing home placement

Wanting "the best"—may mean the family has an agenda that needs to be inquired about

Dissatisfaction with nursing home, staff, doctor, patient care, costs, medications, illness, roommate, and so on

Internal family disagreements

Primary care physician–centered reasons

Lack of response to medical treatments—physician may conclude that symptoms must be psychiatric

Patient noncompliance with medication or other treatments

Nursing staff or administration complaints about the patient to the primary care physician

Nursing home–centered reasons

Requests from consulting pharmacist to bring treatment into OBRA compliance

Changes of administration that lead to changes of nursing home policy

Staff discontent or conflict, which may lead to high turnover

Other reasons

Legal matters (e.g., determination of testamentary capacity)

Financial issues, which may lead to changes in the relationship between the resident and the facility

Situational factors (e.g., a move or contemplated move)

Written Request for a Consultation

The primary care physician's request must be made in writing. Documentation must use the facility's order forms and could include an account of the patient's psychiatric symptoms. At the very least, this information should be listed in the "referral reason" section of the consultation form. Justification of medical necessity in psychiatry can be problematic. Improving the patient's level of functioning and preventing dangerous behavior are two important factors that may underlie medical necessity for a psychiatric consultation. The psychiatrist may avoid unfavorable third-party payer review if he or she documents the referral reasons carefully. Consultation for assistance in custodial care would be difficult to justify to a third-party payer. For example, a patient who is admitted to a facility and has a concomitant mental illness that is stable on a medication regimen would not need a psychiatric consultation for "review of meds."

Expectations of the Primary Care Physician

If the psychiatrist has developed a working relationship with the primary care physician, he or she may know what that physician expects. It may be a single consultation with recommendations made in writing and discussed verbally, or it may be a request for ongoing psychiatric management of the case. This understanding should be clear and explicit in order for the relationship to work well. Ascertainment of the primary care physician's expectations may require extra attention if a working relationship has not been established.

Prior Permission

The consultation's effectiveness is often compromised when the patient or family has not been informed of the referral prior to the psychiatrist's first visit. Ideally the psychiatrist or someone representing him or her should have involved the patient and the family in discussions before the consultation.

Facility Notification

The nursing home should be notified of the psychiatrist's scheduled time of arrival and of the patient to be seen. If the patient's cognition is intact, he or she should be informed of the time scheduled for the visit so that the visit is not an unexpected intrusion. Dropping in at the patient's bedside unannounced may be unwelcome and unproductive. By inviting a family member to be available to provide information, to have an opportunity to ask questions, and with whom to discuss recommendations, the psychiatrist can save time, to say nothing of how this approach can facilitate acceptance of recommendations.

Written Authorization Before Billing

Medicare billing requires a one-time signed authorization executed by the patient or someone acting on the patient's behalf.

Gathering Information

Establishing in an efficient manner a database on a nursing home resident requires a procedure that varies somewhat from that followed in the psychiatrist's office or the hospital. A nursing home staff member who is familiar with the patient may not be readily available, and although a clinical chart is available in a skilled nursing facility, the information in it is arranged in a way that may be unfamiliar to the psychiatrist who is used to working with clinical charts in the hospital.

Clinical Records

It requires time and a concerted effort to look through the patient's chart to find enough clues about how the current problem developed, especially when the psychiatrist is unfamiliar with the facility. A major limitation is that the chart on the unit generally has been culled from information more than a few months old, and extra effort is needed to obtain and study old records that have been filed away. The following sections describe the specific items the psychiatrist should look for.

Minimum Data Set

The Minimum Data Set is a standardized database that provides basic information in checklist format (see Chapter 4). It is updated quarterly and is mandatory for all residents of skilled nursing facilities. It provides a succinct if somewhat sterile record of the patients' problems and limitations.

History and Physical Examination

The patient's history and physical examination report often provides only rudimentary information such as past diagnoses; however, this report is central to the examination of the nursing home resident. It enables the psychiatrist to understand the patient's medical status, including past and current illnesses and treatments. Failure to consider and understand this information can lead to inappropriate recommendations.

Social History

The patient's social history may be the only available source in the record that provides some information about the patient's past, which is important for understanding the context of the current behavior.

Nursing Notes, Vital Signs, and Record of Problem Behavior

Nursing notes, while highly variable, may provide descriptions of disturbed behavior that are essential for understanding the current problem. Any persistent problem behavior should have been recorded in a format that permits the frequency of the behaviors to be evaluated. Behavioral interventions may be noted, but they are inherently more difficult to describe. Recent general medicine problems, including weight changes, are particularly important to note. For patients who have resided at the facility for a long time, old information will have been removed from the patient's chart, and in order to obtain a better picture of the patient's past behaviors the psychiatrist may need to obtain such information from the record room.

Order Sheets and Physicians' Notes

The medications used in the past few months can usually be identified in the order sheets, which may also provide a written rationale for why the medications were given. Efforts to address behavioral issues with medication can therefore be deduced from this record. When physicians' notes coincide with the order dates, they may provide a more detailed explanation.

Medication Administration Records

Several months of medication administration records (MARs) can generally be found in the patient's chart, but the current month's MAR is usually kept in a separate place for the convenience of the nurses who administer the medications. The MAR should be sought in order to obtain an objective record of how behaviors have been addressed with medication in the past few weeks and also to note any new medications being used. Failure to see the current MAR frequently results in errors and off-target recommendations.

Laboratory Reports

Laboratory reports should be scanned for any abnormalities and also may provide a record of drug levels.

Special Reports and Other Records

Cognitive or other psychological tests (e.g., the Mini-Mental State Exam) are often administered to patients at regular intervals. Hospital discharge records tend to provide a more thorough data set and may be present in the patient's chart. The psychiatrist should note the presence of legal documents such as a durable power of attorney or guardianship, along with the name of the person holding such authority.

Patient Interview

The patient interview in the nursing home is like a home visit insofar as it introduces a number of variables not present in the hospital or office setting. The environment in which the interview is conducted may be quite unpredictable and often suboptimal, requiring accommodation to be made. The psychiatrist will need to adjust his or her routine from one facility to another, because what is possible and desirable in one will be unworkable in another. It is usually helpful when a nursing home staff member can accompany the psychiatrist, but one may not always be available unless such a routine has been established with the facility. At a minimum, a suitable chair or chairs should be available in a location that is quiet enough and private enough to permit the psychiatrist to visit with the patient at some leisure. A patient's hearing impairment will often be an issue, and the psychiatrist may find it useful to carry an amplification device.

Introduction

Although respectfulness is an important issue at the first meeting with a patient, it is particularly important with the elderly, who have almost universally suffered a loss of status. Consequently they are addressed less respectfully as a matter of course, in ways that often only they are aware of. The psychiatrist can prevent angry rebuffs if this matter is attended to carefully. For some older patients, being seen by a psychiatrist for the first time in their lives may seem to be an unacceptable insult. In most cases it is helpful for the psychiatrist to stress his or her medical identity and broach the specialty identification only if the question is raised directly. Deliberate misleading of the patient will compound the problem.

Chief Complaint

It is usually best to ask the patient about his or her chief complaint first, even though in cases of behavioral disturbance the consultation is generally requested in response to the problems others are having with the patient's behavior. This approach permits the psychiatrist to hear about the problem from the patient's point of view, to the extent that the patient is aware of it. It shifts the focus from what to do about the resident's problem to what to do for the patient to ameliorate the problem.

History of Present Illness

The patient's history of psychiatric illness and the course of the current disorder should be ascertained as well as possible, but the patient with a behavioral sign or symptom may lack the objectivity if not the cognitive capacity to describe it clearly. It is especially important to be alert to perceived environmental stressors, because behavioral disturbance so often is the final common pathway for what is experienced as intolerable distress. There may be many reasons for that distress, and evaluation of the severity of the various reasons is essential to addressing it. Some sources of problems are impossible to eliminate, but for others remedies may have been overlooked and can therefore be addressed. Understanding the present illness means identifying as clearly as possible the causes of the distress fueling the behavioral disturbance.

Mental Status Examination

The problem behaviors that triggered the consultation may or may not be evident at the time of the visit. The patient's awareness of the problem, and the presence and severity of cognitive impairment, will to a large extent determine the manner in which the mental status examination is performed. At one end of the spectrum the examination will be much the same as with a younger outpatient, but if the patient has advanced dementia, little more than observation will be possible. Observation is particularly important when interviewing the elderly, who may not be able to, or may not choose to, communicate dysphoria verbally. Individuals older than 50 years grew up in a decidedly different environment with regard to how feelings and emotions were regarded and discussed. The language and stigma associated with emotional disturbance were quite different many years ago.

In many patients, perceptual distortions in the form of hallucinations accompany behavioral disturbance. These distortions are a common manifestation of delirium and may also represent adverse effects of prescribed medications, particularly in patients with Parkinson's disease. Hallucinations are more common in the presence of impaired hearing or sight, presumably because of sensory deprivation. Elicitation of such symptoms is best done indirectly with questions such as,

"Have you seen or heard any disturbing things lately that others have not?"

Cognitive distortions in the form of delusions are often a secondary manifestation of impairment, with the delusions becoming progressively less organized as the dementia advances. When delusions are very elaborate, dementia is mild or completely absent, and it may be difficult to determine readily whether dementia is part of the etiology. This is where formal memory tests can help to make the differentiation, if the patient is cooperative. The psychiatrist should note the patient's thought content and preoccupations, particularly because such observations can point to potential remedies for the problem.

Cognitive impairment is usually a factor in behavioral disturbances. Such impairment should be tested by means that are appropriate for the patient's current level of functioning without being unnecessarily intrusive. The psychiatrist can soften the impact of this intrusion by using a supportive manner. Questions about temporal orientation can be introduced by a question such as, "Do you keep track of the time?" Maintenance of an acceptable social facade is very important for persons with dementia, and an attempt to force the patient into a demonstration of his or her breaking point should not be undertaken lightly. We term the inability to maintain this social veneer as *behavioral disturbance,* and we should not test it without regard to the patient's sensibilities, just as we are careful when eliciting physical pain.

Affective disturbance (e.g., irritability, dysphoria, flat or labile affect) is present almost by definition in behavioral problems, because one or more of these disturbances usually are underlying factors in behavioral disturbance. When not present the disturbed behavior is usually more sporadic and the result of specific environmental factors.

The psychiatrist should note the patient's psychomotor activity, including the daily pattern of change in the patient's activity level. This can follow a diurnal pattern, or it may be sporadic, possibly the result of identifiable environmental triggers.

Stressors that may precipitate the disturbed behavior may not be easy to identify if the patient cannot give direct answers to questions as a result of cognitive loss or lack of insight. It is helpful to find out what things displease or distress the patient, in order to determine precipitants of the disturbed behavior. The patient's response will also provide information about his or her coping style, strengths, and weaknesses. Such information can point to accommodations that can be made to eliminate a precipitant of the problem behavior. The rules and regimentation of the nursing home can produce irritation that is particularly distressing to some residents. Often the resident's behavior is a protest that is communicated imperfectly and therefore is not understood or responded to by the nursing home staff. Another question that must always be addressed is whether the patient's behavior is a way of communicating pain or other physical discomfort.

Behavior Inventory

If the psychiatrist observes the problem behavior, such as calling out incessantly, he or she can test interventions to modify the behavior. The results of such interventions can supplement reports of nursing home staff members' efforts. The use of standardized methods of monitoring the level and type of behavioral disturbance enables more reliable evaluation of the effect of interventions and provides a more sophisticated measure of the extent of the presenting problem.

Cohen-Mansfield has classified behavioral agitation in a manner that helps psychiatrists to document it more discretely. She defines agitation broadly as "inappropriate behavior that is unrelated to unmet needs or confusion per se" (Cohen-Mansfield and Billig 1986). The Cohen-Mansfield Agitation Inventory (CMAI) lists 29 problem behaviors, grouped into four categories according to the types of interventions most useful in managing them: 1) aggressive behavior, 2) physically nonaggressive behavior, 3) verbally agitated behavior, and 4) hiding/hoarding behavior (Table 2–2). A monitoring system can be instituted using the CMAI to track the frequency of the behaviors over a period of time, both before and after various interventions.

Interviewing Collateral Sources

Nursing Home Staff

To augment the patient's records and information obtained from the patient interview, the psychiatrist should gather observations from other staff members, for example, a nurse, a social worker, or other staff member designated to be in touch with the psychiatrist. A designated contact at a frequently visited nursing home can be a useful liaison with the staff and the family. The psychiatrist also may want to encourage the staff member to voice opinions, because if the opinions are at odds with the psychiatrist's recommendations, the chances of success are diminished considerably. Whenever possible, differences should be worked through before a recommendation is made.

Family Members

If a family member is not present during the consultation, the psychiatrist may find that telephone contact is useful at the time of the consultation, not only to obtain information but also to develop a relationship that will enlist the family's support in the interventions that are recommended. The family's attitude toward the psychiatrist and the family's level of sophistication can vary dramatically. Assessment of what the family can understand and approve of, before an intervention is recommended, is often crucial to a successful outcome.

Physicians and Other Professionals

Direct contact with a physician who has known the patient provides professional perspective. This physician may not always be the one who requested the consultation. The psychiatrist should note what is currently being done to address the patient's behavioral problem, because this information may provide clues about why current efforts are not successful. Depending on the circumstances, it may also be useful to contact the patient's clergyman or clergywoman to clarify issues from the past. The patient's attorney may also be an important person to contact if the patient's competency is an issue.

Table 2–2. Cohen-Mansfield Agitation Inventory (grouped according to type of behavior)

Aggressive	Physically nonaggressive	Verbally agitated	Hiding/hoarding
Hitting	Pacing	Cursing	Handling things inappropriately
Kicking	Inappropriate robing or disrobing	Constant requests for attention	Hiding things
Grabbing	Spitting	Repetitive sentences or questions	Hoarding things
Pushing	Trying to get to a different place	Making strange noises	
Throwing things	Intentional falling	Screaming	
Biting	Negativism	Complaining	
Scratching	Eating inappropriate substances	Making verbal sexual advances	
Hurting oneself or others	Performing repetitious mannerisms		
Tearing things	General restlessness		
Physical sexual advances			

Source. Adapted from Cohen-Mansfield et al. 1989.

Diagnosis

The diagnostic formulation should address the multiaxial components in the elderly nursing home resident much the same as it does in the younger ambulatory patient. Although identifying DSM-IV diagnoses is necessary and important, a conceptualization of the health of the resident's entire internal and external environment is necessary. The most immediate component of the "family system" the patient relates to is the nursing home, and because it is a relatively new addition to the constellation, significant relationship problems are usually present. Because the patient is less able to verbally communicate these stressors they are correspondingly underrated, delegitimatized, and just overlooked. Family members may try to step into the breach, but they may also distort the communication, especially when the family has had problems. Thus in what might otherwise be a fairly straightforward, treatable case of depression, either the patient or the family may be reluctant to accept the idea of a psychiatric illness.

To arrive at an accurate diagnostic formulation, the psychiatrist ideally weighs all factors—biological, psychological, and social—and assigns each the appropriate significance.

Treatment Formulation and Recommendations

Although we would like to be able to find the "magic bullet" that will solve the patient's problem in one try, the causes of disturbed behavior are in most cases too complex to permit such an easy solution. Pharmacotherapeutic interventions alone are usually insufficient. Quite often they play only an adjunctive role in support of other types of treatment, which should not be omitted in the recommendations.

The psychiatrist's manner of communicating his or her recommendations is a crucial element of successful treatment. All interested parties should be involved in this process so that they are committed to having the recommendations carried out.

Range of Interventions

An exclusive emphasis on medication may compromise the energy with which other interventions are pursued. The value of nonpharmacologic interventions may be lost if they are not addressed specifically in the psychiatrist's report.

Environmental factors may be a sensitive issue for the facility, particularly if the naming of deficiencies implies blaming the nursing home staff or administration. The psychiatrist is in a position to address perceived deficiencies and problems with the nursing home staff. Although mindful and sympathetic to the constraints under which the staff may work, the psychiatrist should be the patient's advocate.

Various social factors, such as family conflict, can be important precipitants of the patient's behavioral disturbance, and these factors should be discussed with the family and others to the extent possible rather than discussing them only with the patient. Often the social services director can be helpful in making the necessary contacts.

Psychological issues can be addressed with psychotherapy when the patient's cognition is adequate and he or she is able to respond to verbal interaction. Adjustment to losses is a ubiquitous problem, particularly for new residents in long-term care facilities. Preparation for the future is always difficult, but preparation for disability and confinement is often neglected. Whether the psychiatrist conducts the psychotherapy or refers the patient elsewhere will depend on the psychiatrist's preference. By being able to provide psychotherapy along with other interventions, the psychiatrist spares the patient the need to learn to relate to yet another caregiver. Group activities conducted by the nursing home staff can play a significant part in addressing psychological issues and can be geared to the needs of individual residents.

Behavioral interventions require explanation and teaching and usually require the help of nurses and nurse assistants to implement them. Based on the inventory of disturbed behaviors and their severity, the psychiatrist can decide on a strategy for treatment and how it might be implemented, along with a monitoring process to assess its effectiveness. David Smith (1995) summarized the types of behavioral interventions that are used for various behavioral disturbances. The physician can reinforce the use of these techniques by practicing them in the presence of those who are with the patient more of the time. Generally many of the nursing home staff members will be more experienced in the use of these interventions. The psychiatrist can play an influential role by encouraging the development of that experience and expertise, and the psychiatrist becomes even more influential as he or she pursues an ongoing working relationship with the staff. Pharmaceutical interventions can be an additional tool that becomes more effective when it is placed in a proper perspective alongside behavioral interventions.

The nursing home staff generally expect the psychiatrist to recommend medication after examining the patient, because that is seen as the psychiatrist's area of expertise. The psychiatrist may be reluctant to disappoint this expectation. The psychiatrist who always prescribes medication may eventually encounter a credibility problem, so that he or she receives no requests for consultation unless, in the opinion of the individual initiating the consultation, they involve the definite need for medication. In presenting the recommendations to the patient, the family, the primary care physician, or the nursing home staff, the psychiatrist should address the entire range of interventions and should temper expectations about medications according to the psychiatrist's estimation of how effective they may be within the context of the complete management program.

If the psychiatrist considers a medication trial to be worthwhile, he or she should convey the prognosis and the rationale for this trial. A good strategy involves outlining a series of trials in order of preference and discussing the merits of each agent, including the symptoms they target. In this way, if the first intervention is not entirely satisfactory, the psychiatrist has not "struck out" and may be permitted to proceed to the next strategy on the list, all the while observing and reinforcing the behavioral interventions being undertaken to alleviate the problem. All interested parties will need to be kept informed, and the psychiatrist will discover by trial and error the amount of energy required to achieve a degree of consensus. Time spent on the problem will be rewarded, but it is necessary to learn during each trial at what locus this scarce commodity can be most potently applied. Certainly neglect of any of the more critical contacts will result in negative feedback and may require the psychiatrist to spend much time on damage control.

Hospitalization or another type of transfer may become necessary if the facility's resources are insufficient to meet the patient's needs or if the staff can no longer manage the patient's behavior. The psychiatrist must be alert to signs from the staff that this point has been reached and must be able to expeditiously arrange for hospitalization. Other interested parties, including the family and the primary care physician, need to be involved in this decision. Depending on the circumstances, the primary care physician may admit the patient, with the psychiatrist offering to consult. The more common arrangement, when an acute medical problem is not present, is for the psychiatrist to assume responsibility for the patient's care in the hospital and consult with the primary care physician as necessary.

Sometimes the resident, the family, or the facility desires a transfer. The nursing home is under an obligation to furnish adequate notice, and avoid unlawful discrimination, before discharging a resident. The psychiatrist can play a useful role as an independent facilitator when there are disputes to see if differences can be resolved. If the problem cannot be resolved, it is helpful if the psychiatrist can broker a separation that will satisfy everyone's interests. This can minimize the possibility of legal action while ensuring that the resident's rights are protected.

As the psychiatrist proceeds, he or she should consider the psychodynamics of the individual patient, the family, and the nursing home staff and the working relationship he or she has with the primary care physician. The patient's previous experiences with doctors and medications and his or her inherent belief system about psychiatric treatment are powerful determinants of the outcomes of the psychiatrist's interventions.

Indications for Pharmacotherapy

Acute Agitation

Agitation is the behavioral problem most often brought to the attention of the psychiatrist. Because of the resident's distress and the disruptive effect that agitation has on the nursing home, this is a problem that should and usually does evoke a response. The threat of, if not the actual development of, combativeness adds an element that can compromise the staff's response and safety.

Nursing staff are expected, under Health Care Financing Administration regulations, to respond to agitation by initiating behavioral interventions and, only if these fail, to consider the use of other methods such as drugs or restraints. Restraints are not acceptable as an ongoing management strategy, and some nursing homes have prohibited their use entirely, both because of the dehumanizing effect of their use and because they have not been shown to be effective in reducing injury.

If the primary care physician has requested an immediate psychiatric consultation with a new patient, the psychiatrist may be pressured to prescribe medication before he or she can perform a thorough, face-to-face evaluation. Before prescribing any agent, the psychiatrist must consider the altered pharmacokinetics and pharmacodynamics of the various agents used in the elderly. The majority of experts recommend that in an emergency a conventional high-potency antipsychotic be used to treat agitation ("Treatment of agitation" 1998). The anticholinergic effects of these drugs may aggravate confusion caused by delirium, and the patient is at increased risk for falls resulting from the hypotensive effects of such medications in the elderly. Some experts prefer to use a short-acting benzodiazepine such as lorazepam, particularly when anxiety is prominent. The psychiatrist must pay attention to the potential for adverse effects, notably ataxia, which increases the risk of falls. Paradoxical excitement may also occur in a small percentage of patients. Some clinicians may alternate lorazepam and haloperidol in intractable situations. The new generation of antipsychotic medications provides an alternative that avoids many of the problems encountered with the traditional agents. As evidence of their efficacy in acute situations accumulates, and they become available in parenteral form, the newer antipsychotics may become the agents of choice. Table 2–3 summarizes the pharmacotherapeutic agents used to treat dementia associated with agitation. The different presentations are described in the sections that follow.

The psychiatrist should examine the patient as soon as possible to evaluate the effect of the emergency intervention and to determine the nature and potential causes of the agitation. It is particularly important not to overlook pain as a possible cause of agitation, especially when dementia is advanced and the patient has lost the ability to communicate effectively. Appropriate analgesia should be administered when pain is suspected.

The most frequent cause of sporadic, episodic agitation in patients with dementia is a resistive reaction to personal care, such as toileting and bathing. Ongoing use of medication to control such reactions is generally not warranted, but in some individuals it has been helpful to give a short-acting benzodiazepine routinely one-half hour before a bath or shower.

Recurring Agitation

Agitation can become chronic and resistant to behavioral interventions, possibly because behavioral interventions have not been instituted promptly enough. As the dementia patient's level of cognitive impairment increases, he or she is subject to catastrophic reactions that are the result of excess demand on a limited cognitive capacity. Although their usefulness in ameliorating behavioral symptoms has yet to be demonstrated, cholinesterase inhibitors, such as donepezil, may be able to bring about improvement by increasing

the patient's cognitive capacity or otherwise reducing the patient's tendency to become agitated.

It is useful to observe the patient's behavior closely to determine how the symptoms can be targeted successfully with medication, taking into account the adverse effects (e.g., hypotension, ataxia, sedation) to which the patient may be most vulnerable.

If evidence indicates that the agitation is driven by delusional preoccupation or disturbing hallucinations, the psychiatrist should start the patient on an antipsychotic medication. The phenothiazines and other older agents have a high incidence of adverse effects in the elderly. Tardive dyskinesia occurs much more often in the elderly with dementia than in the general population and can develop after just a few weeks. The novel antipsychotic agents are promising and avoid many of the extrapyramidal side effects and much of the risk of tardive dyskinesia. Studies have shown risperidone to be effective for this condition; however, because the novel antipsychotics are more costly, resistance may be encountered from those paying for them.

If the patient has agitation with flight of ideas and hyperactivity, the psychiatrist can prescribe an antimanic agent that can be used even in the absence of a history of bipolar disorder. Because the therapeutic index of lithium is quite low, and because of the reduced kidney clearance and greater danger of toxic reactions in the elderly, it has become commonplace to use divalproex or carbamazepine to reduce hyperactivity.

Buspirone has been shown to be effective when anxiety is prominent. Regular long-term use of benzodiazepines, even the shorter-acting agents, is usually not justified. The eventual development of tolerance frequently results in a recurrence of agitation that worsens when an attempt is made to withdraw the drug, because of a rebound effect. Trazodone in small doses at appropriate times of the day is often used to provide mild sedation.

If agitation is accompanied by dysphoria and irritability, depression is the most likely cause, and the agitation should be treated as such. For immediate sedation, trazodone can be used alone or in combination with a selective serotonin

Table 2–3. Pharmacotherapeutic agents used to treat dementia associated with agitation

Type of presentation	Initial agent
Acute agitation with combativeness	Neuroleptics, benzodiazepines, analgesics
Agitation with delusions or hallucinations	Neuroleptics
Agitation with flight of ideas or hyperactivity	Valproate, carbamazepine
Agitation with anxiety	Buspirone, trazodone
Agitation with dysphoria or irritability	Antidepressants

reuptake inhibitor (SSRI) at appropriate times of the day in titrated doses to ameliorate the agitation more immediately. Nefazodone or mirtazapine combine a degree of sedation with good antidepressant effect.

Depression

Depression is usually manifested by apathy, irritability, and dysphoria, symptoms that are often quite responsive to pharmacotherapy. Electroconvulsive therapy is also a consideration for the elderly, especially if the patient's distress is extreme or the depression is refractory to antidepressants.

Apathy often is not considered a behavioral disturbance because it is less likely to trouble the people around patients who exhibit it. It is one of the most commonly encountered disturbances characteristic of Alzheimer's dementia, and it can be a sign of depression. A patient's apathy may not be brought to the attention of the psychiatrist unless he or she has a working relationship with nursing staff who are also alert to this problem. Secondary to apathy may be poor nutritional intake and accelerated physical decline with accompanying loss of ability to independently perform activities of daily living. In any one case it is difficult to judge whether such behavior will respond to antidepressant medication, but because these medications have a relative lack of adverse effects, a therapeutic trial is frequently indicated. Sometimes a small dose of methylphenidate is given to increase the patient's activity level.

Irritability is a characteristic of depression that often is not identified correctly. Because it tends to elicit negative feelings, staff may regard irritability as a characterological problem and not bring it to the attention of the psychiatrist. It is particularly important that the psychiatrist makes an effort to deal sensitively with patients who exhibit a "prickly" manner, in order to persuade these patients to take the risk to talk about feelings.

Dysphoria alone is more likely to come to the psychiatrist's attention, particularly if the patient expresses feelings of not wanting to live.

The psychiatrist must consider the possibility of interactions between antidepressants and other medications, particularly with monoamine oxi-

dase inhibitors, which may be used in Parkinson's disease. The inhibition of P450 liver enzymes by various antidepressant agents must also be considered. Although the SSRIs and other newer agents have largely displaced the tricyclic antidepressants, there may still be a place for nortriptyline or desipramine, particularly when the patient or family members resist paying the price of newer medications still under patent. The psychiatrist will often encounter the older agents, particularly small doses of amitriptyline because of its touted effect as an analgesic. The psychiatrist should consider replacing amitriptyline with effective doses of nortriptyline that can target the symptoms of depression.

Documentation

The psychiatrist should document his or her findings in a legible written report that is sent to the physician who requested the consultation and added to the patient's record. The psychiatrist should keep another copy for reference—for example, in case of telephone inquiries about the patient or to justify the billing code used. Because multiple copies may be needed, dictation or typing of the initial report is preferable. This also establishes the psychiatrist as someone who is serious and careful about work in the long-term care setting. Having the record available in an electronic form makes it useful for handling telephone inquiries expeditiously.

Continuation of Treatment

The attending physician's wishes with regard to the psychiatrist's ongoing management of a behavioral problem should be clarified. Otherwise, the primary care physician may not know when to step in to address new or ongoing problems. If called by the nursing staff in an emergency, the primary care physician may then take over in the absence of a clearly defined understanding of whether the psychiatrist is still monitoring the case. Ideally the psychiatrist should continue to be available to monitor the treatment as long as required to address the behavioral problem. Timing of succeeding visits needs to be planned, and the nursing staff should know how to contact the psychiatrist with questions or new and unexpected developments. Special instructions about the circumstances that should trigger a call can be written on the order sheet. Even if a patient is stable, a maximum time period between visits should be established for as long as the psychiatrist is following the case. If further visits appear unnecessary—either because the patient is asymptomatic and no psychotropic medications are being used or because it is deemed appropriate to ask the primary care physician to assume responsibility for monitoring the treatment—then this should be stated formally.

As the dementia progresses in a particular patient the clinical picture will change, and in time medications may not be needed. When it is no longer clear that the agent being used is effective, the psychiatrist should initiate a gradual withdrawal. Federal regulations governing nursing facilities mandate withdrawal trials of benzodiazepines and antipsychotics in the case of dementia diagnoses at least once every 6 months, unless documentation gives an adequate rationale for continuing the medication. Failure to do so puts the nursing home at risk of being cited for noncompliance.

The psychiatrist is usually called into the nursing home initially to deal with a particular crisis, but in order to play a useful role, he or she must be able to shift from crisis intervention, to treatment, to prevention. This involves establishing a therapeutic alliance, which is as important in nursing homes as it is in other settings. Here the alliance includes the nursing home staff, the primary care physician, the family, and the patient. When this alliance is in place the psychiatrist in the nursing home can provide a valuable service not only to the individual nursing home resident but also to the entire system devoted to the care of that resident.

References

Cohen-Mansfield J, Billig N: Agitated behaviors in the elderly, I: a conceptual review. J Am Geriatr Soc 34:711–721, 1986

Cohen-Mansfield J, Marx MS, Rosenthal AS: A description of agitation in a nursing home. J Gerontol 44:M77–84, 1989

Smith DA: Geriatric Psychopathology: Behavioral Intervention as First Line Treatment. Providence, RI, Manisses Communications Group, 1995

Treatment of agitation in older persons with dementia. Postgrad Med (special report), April 1998

Chapter 3

Sexuality in the Nursing Home

Sex and Aging

Although sexual function is often a vital part of late life, a number of physiologic changes occur with aging that are important to consider in understanding sexual expression. For example, a man's ejaculation control may improve as he ages. Pleasure continues with orgasm, although older men may require a longer refractory period before erection occurs again. For older women, declining estrogen production causes shrinking of the uterus, thinning of vaginal mucosa, and diminished vaginal lubrication. Despite these physical changes, interest and pleasure in sex continues for both sexes well into the later years of life (Richardson and Lazur 1995).

Although society often views sexuality in older adults as a taboo or nonexistent subject, many older adults living in institutional settings continue to express an interest in sex. Bretschneider and McCoy (1988) surveyed residents of 10 California life-care communities and found that 70% of men and 50% of women had frequent thoughts of wanting a close or intimate relationship with the opposite sex (Bretschneider and McCoy 1988). The most frequent sexual behaviors included touching their partner, masturbation, and sexual intercourse. Of the residents surveyed, 53% of men and 25% of women had regular sex partners.

In a nursing home setting, views on sexuality may become increasingly limited (Mulligan and Modigh 1991). In a survey of nursing home residents' views of sexuality, Kaas (1978) found that 61% of residents did not feel sexually attractive.

Wasow and Loeb (1979) found that residents of a Wisconsin nursing home believed sexual activity was appropriate for other elderly people in their nursing home; however, they were not often personally involved because of lack of opportunity. Most residents endorsed having sexual feelings and thoughts.

Addressing Sexual Behavior: Staff Attitudes, Patient Approach, and Treatment

Nursing home staff may ask the psychiatrist to evaluate nursing home patients for sexual behaviors they deem inappropriate. Szaz (1983) found that nursing staff of a 400-bed facility estimated that 25% of their male residents demonstrated "problematic" sexual behavior. This behavior included sex talk (using "dirty" language), implied sexual behavior (viewing pornographic material), and sexual acts (grabbing staff, masturbating).

The psychiatrist may be asked to evaluate inappropriate sexual behaviors, and exploring with the staff their own attitudes toward sexuality in late life may be a first step toward developing an effective intervention. Staff can benefit greatly from education about the myths and taboos of elder sexuality, physiologic changes in sexual functioning with aging, the role of sexuality in health maintenance, mechanisms for compensating for physical disabilities, and the establishment of firm personal boundaries with patients (Steinke 1997).

The nursing home psychiatrist is also in an excellent position to educate the staff about the neurophysiologic deterioration associated with dementia and the effect of such changes on the patient's behavior. By explaining that cortical changes associated with dementia may be the cause of the patient's disinhibited sexual language or behaviors, the psychiatrist will assist nursing home staff in understanding and integrating these behaviors into a medical disease model.

Staff attitudes may also be challenged by alternative sexual relationships. Little information is currently available on homosexuality in the nursing home. Some figures suggest that 8%–10% of the population have alternative sexual lifestyles (Deevy 1990). Lyder (1994) pointed out that if this percentage is accurate, then dealing with homosexual, bisexual, or gender identity issues presents another virtually unexplored area for the staff.

By allowing an open discussion of the staff's attitudes toward sexuality in late life, the psychiatrist may diffuse the staff's own anxieties and allow them to depersonalize a patient's inappropriate verbal comments or touches. The psychiatrist can act as a role model by giving residents who make sexual statements firm but kind feedback on the inappropriate nature of their language or behavior. Table 3–1 provides suggestions for addressing these behaviors.

Likewise, by discussing the role of masturbation in sexual functioning and the need for patient privacy, the psychiatrist may help move the staff's initial shock reactions toward understanding of this behavior (Letters to the Editor 1997). Some facilities have also developed "intimacy groups" to help residents deal with their sexuality in an institutional setting (Tunstull and Henry 1996). Through education, the psychiatrist may help prevent the labeling of patients as "dirty old men" or "perverts."

Pharmacologic approaches to managing inappropriate behavior have included treatment with psychotropic medications and estrogens. A small series of case reports over the past 10 years has suggested that antiandrogens may diminish sexu-

Table 3–1. Approaches to sexual behavior

Openly discuss sexual needs with the resident and partner

Provide the resident with privacy for sexual activities (shut door, pull curtain)

Educate resident and staff about age-related sexual changes

Avoid the use of negative subjective labels while discussing the resident

Encourage the use of touch (e.g., hand holding, hugging) and one-to-one visits during care to provide intimacy and fulfill the resident's needs for physical and emotional closeness

Attend to the resident's grooming and personal hygiene to maintain his or her attractiveness and self-esteem

Encourage the staff not to "overreact" to sexual comments or behaviors; instead provide neutral verbal feedback on inappropriateness and leave the room

ally aggressive behavior in men. Cooper (1987, 1988) used medroxyprogesterone acetate to diminish disruptive sexual behavior in four demented male patients. Likewise, Kyomen et al. (1991a, 1991b) found that conjugated estrogen and diethylstilbestrol decreased aggression in two male patients. However, double-blind clinical trials of antiandrogen therapies are currently lacking in the literature. Little clinical evidence suggests that these medications eliminate target inappropriate sexual behaviors, suggesting that clinicians should rely on a behavioral or environmental approach to address sexuality issues.

A number of medications can adversely affect sexual functioning. These include psychotropic medications (e.g., neuroleptics, selective serotonin reuptake inhibitors, tricyclic antidepressants, monoamine oxidase inhibitors), antihypertensives, digoxin, narcotics, anticonvulsants, cimetidine, and metoclopramide (Richardson and Lazur 1995).

Sexuality and Cognition

When spouses of demented patients place them in the nursing home, a loss of shared intimacy may occur. The caregiver's desire for sexual intimacy may conflict with worries that the patient will not recognize him or her, will make frequent sexual overtures, or will act in a sexually inappropriate manner in public (Davies et al. 1992; Litz et al. 1990).

The nursing home psychiatrist may find that exploring a couple's sexual history and current needs is an important component of an effective treatment plan. Developing a private room for "intimate visits," allowing for overnight visits, and acknowledging a couple's need for closeness are helpful strategies that nursing homes may provide to address the resident's and spouse's sexual needs. Educating the spouse to not over-react to sexually inappropriate statements or behavior is an important role of the psychiatrist. Encouraging privacy, distraction, or gentle re-direction may be alternative strategies to deal with these behaviors.

Occasionally, a situation arises when patients with a compromised cognitive ability to consent to sexual activity express the desire to have sex. This scenario may include sex between cognitively compromised residents or a couple in which one individual is competent to give consent for sex and the other is not. The psychiatrist may be called on to evaluate an individual's judgment-making capacity to consent for sex. Often the "need to protect" a vulnerable patient must be weighed against the patient's cognitive capacities. The cognitive capacities required to understand and desire sex may be very different from those required to manage financial affairs or make major medical decisions. Discussion with surrogate decision makers, such as guardians or those holding powers of attorney, should be an integral part of the psychiatric consultation.

References

Bretschneider JG, McCoy NL: Sexual interest and behavior in healthy 80–102 year olds. Arch Sex Behav 17:109–129, 1988

Cooper AJ: Medroxyprogesterone acetate (MPA) treatment of sexual acting out in men suffering from dementia. J Clin Psychiatry 48:368–370, 1987

Cooper AJ: Medroxyprogesterone acetate (MPA) treatment of sexual acting out in men suffering from organic brain syndrome. Am J Psychiatry 145:1179–1180, 1988

Davies D, Zeiss A, Tinklenberg JR: Til death do us part: intimacy and sexuality in the marriages of Alzheimer's patients. Journal of Psychosocial Nursing 30:5–10, 1992

Deevy S: Older lesbian women and the invisible minority. Journal of Gerontological Nursing 16:35–37, 1990

Kaas MJ: Sexual expression of the elderly in nursing homes. Gerontologist 18:372–378, 1978

Kyomen HH, Kohn D, Wei J: Gender-linked objections to hormonal treatment of aggression in men with dementia. Gerontologist 31:273, 1991a

Kyomen HH, Nobel KW, Wei JY: The use of estrogen to decrease aggressive physical behavior in elderly men with dementia. J Am Geriatr Soc 39:1110–1112, 1991b

Letters to the Editor, Journal of Gerontological Nursing 10:52–55, 1997

Litz BT, Zeiss AM, Davies HD: Sexual concerns of male spouses of female Alzheimer's disease patients. Gerontologist 30:113–116, 1990

Lyder CH: The role of the nurse practitioner in promoting sexuality in the institutionalized elderly. Journal of the American Academy of Nurse Practitioners 6:61–63, 1994

Mulligan T, Modigh A: Sexuality in dependent living situations. Clin Geriatr Med 7:153–160, 1991

Richardson JP, Lazur A: Sexuality in the nursing home patient. Am Fam Physician 51:121–124, 1995

Steinke EE: Sexuality in aging: implications for nursing facility staff. The Journal of Continuing Education in Nursing 28:59–63, 1997

Szaz G: Sexual incidents in an extended care unit for aged men. J Am Geriatr Soc 31:407–411, 1983

Tunstull P, Henry ME: Approaches to resident sexuality. Journal of Gerontological Nursing 6:37–42, 1996

Wasow M, Loeb MB: Sexuality in nursing homes. J Am Geriatr Soc 27:73–79, 1979

Section 2

Regulatory Aspects

*OBRA, the Minimum Data Set, and Other
Regulations That Affect Nursing Home Practice*

Chapter 4

The Minimum Data Set as a Tool for the Psychiatrist

According to the Nursing Home Reform Act of 1987, all Medicaid-certified nursing facilities must record a structured assessment of every resident within 14 days of admission and must record a follow-up assessment quarterly or when the resident's status changes significantly. These structured assessments are designed to identify problems that require further evaluation or management. Facilities are required to demonstrate appropriate follow-up of problems identified in the structured assessment. Surveyors may find nursing homes out of compliance with federal regulations if they fail to do so.

The structured assessment required by federal regulations is called the Resident Assessment Instrument (RAI). The RAI consists of three components: 1) the Minimum Data Set (MDS), an instrument for recording health status, functional status, and health service use, mainly through responses to checklists and multiple-choice items; 2) Resident Assessment Protocols (RAPs), structured approaches to the further assessment of clinical issues identified (triggered) by items on the MDS (RAPs are intended to be a bridge between the MDS assessment and individualized care planning); and 3) Utilization Guidelines, rules regarding when MDS assessments must be done and their relationship to care planning and clinical documentation.

Since June 1998, all nursing homes certified by Medicare and/or Medicaid have been required to submit computerized MDS records to a desig-nated state agency, which in turn transmits the records to the Health Care Financing Administration (HCFA) for archiving. Residents must have MDS assessments regardless of their source of payment. Follow-up assessments are required at least quarterly and whenever a significant change in the resident's status occurs. Annual reassessments use the full MDS form. Routine quarterly assessments use an abbreviated form with fewer items, focusing on symptoms and functional capacities likely to change from quarter to quarter. Those include physical function (activities of daily living [ADLs]), continence, pain, mood, cognition, and behavior.

Since July 1998, Medicare has based payment for skilled nursing facility care on a per diem rate determined by the resident's MDS assessment. A skilled nursing facility resident is assigned to 1 of 44 Resource Utilization Groups (RUGs) based on application of classification rules to 108 specified MDS items. Medicare-funded residents must be assessed on or about day 5, day 14, and days 30, 60, and 90 of their stay in the facility.

HCFA has also funded the development of Quality Indicators (QIs) based on the MDS items. Individual residents may or may not "trigger" particular QIs. As of this writing, there are 30 QIs; examples are the prevalence of falls and the prevalence of pressure ulcers. With HCFA's encouragement, state surveyors increasingly are using QIs to focus their inspections of nursing facilities. Twelve QIs are of particular interest to geriatric psychiatrists: 1) prevalence of problem behavior toward others, 2) prevalence of symptoms of depression, 3) prevalence of depression with no treatment, 4) use of nine or more scheduled medications, 5) incidence of cognitive impairment, 6) prevalence of antipsychotic use in the absence of psychotic and related conditions, 7) prevalence of antipsychotic daily doses in excess of surveyor guidelines, 8) prevalence of any antianxiety or hypnotic use, 9) prevalence of hypnotic use on a scheduled basis of as-needed more than twice in the last week, 10) prevalence of any long-acting benzodiazepine, 11) prevalence of daily restraints, and 12) prevalence of little or no activity.

Some nursing homes fully integrate the MDS and the RAPs into their care planning process. Others comply only with the letter of the law, relying on an MDS nurse to fill out forms for compliance with regulations. Physicians in particular often do not make use of the MDS or participate significantly in its completion. The new payment methodology compels nursing homes to be timely and accurate in their completion of MDS assessments. This makes MDS data more valuable to clinicians of all disciplines. With time, it should increase the integration of the RAI with clinical care.

Mental Health Elements of the MDS

The full MDS form has more than 500 multiple-choice questions and checklist items. It is divided into sections related to different domains, for example, physical functioning and structural problems and mood and behavior patterns. Several sections relate specifically to the resident's mental health, and other sections have individual items that are important to the psychiatrist. The next several sections describe these items as they appear in the MDS, Version 2.0:

Section AB: Demographic Information

Content. This section records where the resident lived in the 5 years before he or she entered the nursing home; whether he or she lived alone; the resident's lifetime occupation, education, and pri-

mary language; and whether the resident has a formal history of mental illness, mental retardation, or developmental disability.

Section AC: Customary Routine

Content. This section records the resident's customary routine during the year before he or she entered the nursing home. For example, did he or she stay up late at night, take naps, have hobbies, get around independently, smoke tobacco, or drink alcohol? It also records the resident's social involvement. For example, did he or she see relatives or friends daily, attend religious services or find strength in faith, have an animal companion, or participate in groups?

Clinical use. By comparing the resident's former routines with the restrictions and opportunities in the nursing home, the psychiatrist can determine how much placement in the home has disrupted the resident's lifestyle and caused a loss of the activities that gave quality to the resident's life. If an admission MDS has little or no information in this section about the resident's customary routine, it raises the concern that the facility's staff does not know the resident very well. Interpersonal problems between residents and staff can arise when the latter do not appreciate the resident's individuality and help the resident preserve it in the institutional environment of the nursing facility.

Section A: Identification and Background Information

Content. This section records the resident's marital status and source of payment for care; his or her status regarding legal responsibility, including guardianship status, durable powers of attorney, and management of financial affairs by family members; and advance medical directives and orders, including living wills, organ donation plans, autopsy requests, and restrictions on treatment (e.g., do not resuscitate; do not hospitalize; restrictions on feeding, medications, or other treatments).

Clinical use. When a resident is not competent but has no guardian, durable power of attorney, or other advance directives, there is a risk of delayed or poor decision making in a time of medical crisis. When a resident appears to be incompetent and does not have an identified substitute decision maker, the psychiatrist should raise the issue with the attending physician and/or nursing staff.

Section B: Cognitive Patterns

Content. This section provides information on the resident's memory and cognitive skills for daily decision making and records any indicators of delirium or recent change in cognitive status.

Clinical use. The memory sections ask very basic questions, such as whether the resident knows he or she is in a nursing home or knows the location of his or her room. As such, these sections screen for gross memory disturbance but are not a substitute for clinical memory testing.

The item on cognitive skills for daily decision making is a global assessment of the resident's executive cognitive function. It is remarkably reliable and valid. "Independence" on this item means the resident's decisions are both consistent and reasonable. Mildly impaired residents have difficulty in new situations only, moderately impaired residents need cues and supervision, and severely impaired residents rarely if ever make decisions.

Indicators of delirium are generally consistent with DSM criteria and are to be based on staff and family observations of the resident's behavior over the past 7 days.

As nursing facility staff typically score them, the MDS delirium items tend to be specific but not sensitive. If *any* signs of delirium are noted on the MDS, the psychiatric consultation should include a reassessment for this problem.

Section C: Communication/ Hearing Patterns

Content. This section records information about the resident's hearing, hearing aid use, alternate communication such as sign language, clarity of speech, ability to understand others, ability to make himself or herself understood, and recent changes in communication or hearing.

Clinical use. This section, while reliable as far as it goes, does not distinguish among causes of impairment. Ear problems are not distinguished from central nervous system problems, nor are laryngeal problems distinguished from aphasia. If problems are identified in this section, the psychiatrist should check the resident's medical record and other data sources for diagnostic information. If significant hearing and communication problems are present, the psychiatrist should make provisions to mitigate them during the evaluation. The psychiatrist should consider whether communication and hearing problems were taken into account during prior evaluations of the resident's memory, mood, and cognition.

Section E: Mood and Behavior Patterns

Content. This section records whether the resident shows the following indications of depression and anxiety: verbal expressions of emotional distress; sleep-cycle problems; sad, apathetic, anxious appearance; or loss of interest. These indications are supplemented by information on the resident's mood persistence and reactivity in the week prior to the assessment and whether the resident's mood has changed in the past 90 days or since the last assessment. This section also records the resident's behavioral symptoms—for example, wandering, verbally abusive behavior, physically abusive behavior, socially inappropriate or disruptive behavior, and resistance to care—and whether behavioral symptoms have changed recently. The frequency of occurrence of behavioral symptoms over the past week is recorded as "not at all," "1–3 days out of 7," "4–6 days out of 7," or "daily."

Clinical use. The mood sections parallel DSM criteria for major depression, although the precise wording would not permit a direct correlation with any DSM diagnosis. The behavioral section distinguishes between dangerous behavior and that which is merely problematic for the facility. This is particularly important when considering the appropriateness of neuroleptic drugs and physical restraints. Neuroleptic drugs and restraints are not indicated for wandering alone or for benign but socially inappropriate behavior not due to a psychotic disorder.

When behavioral problems do not occur daily, the days on which they do occur provide an initial clue to potential triggers for the behavior. When they occur daily, the first step in identifying triggers would be to determine the time of day or location where the behavioral problems usually take place.

Section F: Psychosocial Well-Being

Content. This section records the resident's sense of initiative and involvement. For example, is he or she at ease doing planned or structured activities; does he or she initiate activities and establish goals, pursue involvement in the life of the facility, or accept invitations into group activities? It also addresses the resident's relationship issues. For example, is the resident unhappy with his or her roommate or with other residents, in conflict with staff, angry with family or friends? Is the resident socially isolated, or has he or she had a recent major loss? Is the resident rigid regarding changes in routines? Is he or she preoccupied with a loss of roles, status, or customary activities and routines?

Clinical use. This section addresses the resident's mental health rather than the symptoms of mental illness. The items on initiative and involvement are a reliable and valid screen for apathy. When apathy is present, diagnostic considerations include depression, parkinsonism, medication side effects (including sedation and akinesia), frontal lobe involvement by neurologic disease, and fatigue due to chronic medical problems. The items on relationships and past roles reflect the interaction between the resident's personality and the present circumstances. Knowing the resident's social and developmental history, the psychiatrist can gauge the relative importance of present circumstances in determining the resident's emotional state. Environmental interventions (e.g., activities, care plans, change in room) and psychotherapy may be needed to address the relationship problems identified in these items.

Section G: Physical Functioning and Structural Problems

Content. This section records a complete assessment of physical ADLs. Of psychiatric importance, a distinction is made between what the resident does independently and what he or she can do with supervision but no physical help.

Clinical use. If a resident can do more with supervision, cueing, and encouragement than he or she does alone, the reasons may include impaired executive function, decreased motivation, apathy, psychosis, or depression. The psychiatric evaluation should emphasize diagnoses and interventions related to the potential recovery of independent function. If a psychotropic drug leads to demonstrable improvement in function, then families, regulators, nurses, and primary care physicians can usually be convinced that its use is appropriate.

Section H: Continence in Last 14 Days

Content. Regarding bowel and bladder function, is the resident continent, usually incontinent, occasionally incontinent, frequently incontinent, or virtually always incontinent? Are there problems with constipation, diarrhea, or fecal impaction? Does the resident have a bladder training program or use catheters or other appliances? Has urinary continence changed in the past 90 days?

Clinical use. Incontinence is one of the reasons that family caregivers offer for eventually opting to place a relative in a nursing home. When incontinence can be corrected, the resident's social options and residential options may improve. This may improve the resident's mood and well-being. Residents with intermittent incontinence are more likely than those with continuous incontinence to have completely reversible problems. Most residents with intermittent incontinence will benefit from a systematic and rigorous evaluation, followed by an appropriate combination of specific medical treatment, adjustment of their medication regimen, dietary changes or fluid restriction, and scheduled toileting.

Incontinence and constipation are relatively common side effects of psychotropic drugs in the nursing home. A frequent scenario is that an anticholinergic drug causes constipation and fecal impaction, which leads to urinary incontinence due to pressure on the bladder by impacted feces. Psychiatrists must ensure that their patients have normal bowel function, by prescribing or recommending bowel regimens when they prescribe drugs that cause constipation. Incontinence that develops on neuroleptic therapy often is an indirect result of extrapyramidal side effects and may be treatable with antiparkinsonian drugs. Urinary retention due to anticholinergic psychotropic drugs can be treated with bethanechol or donepezil. If retention is aggravated by bladder neck obstruction due to prostatic hyperplasia, α-adrenergic blocking drugs may be useful. The key point is that constipation and continence are important risk factors that the psychiatrist should identify before prescribing psychotropic drugs, and these risk factors should be monitored during therapy. The MDS items are useful tools for this purpose.

Section I: Disease Diagnoses

Content. This section records the resident's active medical diagnoses that are thought to be related to his or her present functional status, cognition, mood, behavior, medical treatments, nursing care requirements, or risk of death. These are presented as a checklist, with blanks for filling in additional diagnoses and their ICD-9 codes. Endocrine diagnoses include diabetes, hypothyroidism, and hyperthyroidism. Neuropsychiatric diagnoses include Alzheimer's disease, aphasia, cerebral palsy, stroke, dementia other than Alzheimer's disease, hemiparesis or hemiplegia, multiple sclerosis, paraplegia, Parkinson's disease,

quadriplegia, seizure disorder, transient ischemic attack, and traumatic brain injury. Psychiatric diagnoses include anxiety disorder, depression, bipolar disorder, and schizophrenia.

Clinical use. Facilities vary greatly in how completely and accurately they record disease diagnoses. For example, many facilities do not record dementia diagnoses for most of their cognitively impaired residents. Also, many residents may be treated for depression without the diagnosis being checked in this section. Even when diagnoses are recorded accurately, this section doesn't distinguish between treated and untreated conditions. Nonetheless, the conditions checked can help focus the evaluation on general medical factors causing or contributing to a resident's mental disorder.

Section J: Health Conditions

Content. This section records the resident's symptoms and signs of disease in the past 7 days, such as pain (frequency, intensity, and site), vomiting, fever, edema, and falls and other accidents. Two items of particular psychiatric relevance are hallucinations and unsteady gait.

Clinical use. The presence of hallucinations on the most recent MDS focuses the evaluation on signs of psychosis or delirium. If the resident's gait was unsteady on the most recent MDS assessment, or if the resident has fallen recently, his or her gait should be reevaluated and orthostatic blood pressure checked. Gait disturbance and falls can be a sign of psychotropic drug side effects. Medication can affect gait directly, as do the benzodiazepines and the SSRIs. Other medications affect gait by causing parkinsonism or orthostatic hypotension. When a resident has a gait disturbance, the psychiatrist should address the issue of whether it is due to a psychotropic drug. A well-founded psychiatric opinion that a gait problem is *not* related to a psychotropic drug may prevent the discontinuation of a useful medication.

Review of pain symptoms is crucial in the psychiatric evaluation of the nursing home resident, because pain is highly prevalent and often untreated or ineffectively treated. A resident with dementia may exhibit severe agitation because of pain from osteoarthritis; treatment of the latter with acetaminophen may relieve the agitation. If the resident has a known condition that usually is painful, but no pain symptoms are checked on the MDS, the psychiatrist should consider that cognitive impairment or communication problems may be preventing the resident from expressing pain complaints. Agitation or facial expressions of distress should raise the suspicion that the resident is in pain and should lead the psychiatrist to consider a trial of an analgesic.

Section K: Oral/Nutritional Status

Content. This section records the resident's height and weight, weight change, oral problems, feeding problems, and the facility's approach to these problems.

Clinical use. Documented weight loss with other depressive symptoms should motivate treatment of depression or reconsideration of the treatment if the resident has been on antidepressants for some time. Weight loss as an antidepressant side effect should be considered in residents receiving selective serotonin reuptake inhibitors or bupropion. Oral problems in residents who are taking neuroleptics should trigger a careful assessment for tardive dyskinesia. If a resident with dementia or apathy has a poor oral intake, the psychiatrist should review the circumstances of feeding. Some residents with dementia will eat adequately if cued by their physical and social environment (e.g., in a dining room with other people and appealing food) but not if given a tray of institutional food in their room.

Section N: Activity Pursuit Patterns

Content. This section records the resident's time awake; average time involved in activities; preferred settings of activity; and preferred types of activity, such as playing cards and other games,

participating in arts and crafts, exercising, watching or participating in sports, playing or listening to music, reading or writing, taking trips or going shopping, walking or wheeling outdoors, gardening or looking at plants, watching TV, conversing, or helping others. This section also records whether the resident wants a change in his or her daily routine.

Clinical use. The resident's time awake and active is another valid measure of apathy and an early and objective indicator of drug-induced sedation or akinesia. A low level of activity, in the absence of severe or acute physical illness or advanced dementia, suggests depression, apathy, or drug toxicity or a mismatch of available activities with the resident's abilities and interests. Because inactivity is a major risk factor for cognitive and functional decline, the psychiatrist should identify the specific reasons for a resident's inactivity. Some nursing facilities offer a relatively narrow range of activities, leaving some residents with nothing to do that interests them. The lack of suitably trained staff may provide another barrier to participation in activities; however, nursing homes are obliged by regulations to provide residents with appropriate activities. The consulting psychiatrist in the nursing home has an important role in advocating for residents when a lack of appropriate and interesting activities causes residents to become apathetic and withdrawn.

One of the potential benefits of Alzheimer's special care units is the provision of a wider range of activities that are appropriate for and interesting to cognitively impaired people. When such units engage residents in substantial daily activity, the residents have fewer problems with sleep disturbances, mood disturbances, and behavioral problems. In particular, sufficient engagement in structured activity can reduce wandering, sleep disturbances, and disruptive or socially inappropriate behavior.

Section O: Medications

Content. This section records the number of medications the resident has taken in the past

7 days; whether new medications were introduced in the past 90 days; whether injections are given; and whether the resident receives antipsychotic drugs, anxiolytic drugs, antidepressant drugs, hypnotic drugs, or diuretics.

Clinical use. The MDS item on medication changes in the preceding 90 days can cue the psychiatrist to query staff about recent medication changes and the reasons for them. The medical record will not necessarily contain information about the reasons that medications were changed.

All of the specific medications listed can have a direct or indirect effect on gait and the risk of falling. When several are checked, it suggests that the psychiatrist should formally examine the resident's gait and check for orthostatic hypotension.

Section P: Special Treatments and Procedures

Content. This section begins with a long checklist of special treatments and programs, such as oxygen therapy and hospice care. Of particular importance to the psychiatrist are the items on physical therapy, occupational therapy, speech therapy, and psychological therapy. The section continues with a checklist of interventions for mood, behavioral, and cognitive problems, including symptom evaluation programs, specialist mental health consultation, group therapy, resident-specific environmental changes, and cueing/reorientation programs. This section also records the use of restraints, including bed rails, side rails, trunk restraints, limb restraints, and chairs that prevent the resident from rising; the number of hospital stays and emergency room visits in the past 90 days; and the number of physician visits and orders in the past 2 weeks.

Clinical use. The items on therapies and behavioral interventions enable the psychiatrist to determine what approaches have been tried for the resident's problem. The restraint items enable the psychiatrist to determine whether the facility has gotten the resident out of restraints or into restraints, and whether restraints are an ongoing

part of the resident's treatment. Current thinking in geriatrics is that the long-term use of physical restraints is virtually never justified.

Section Q: Discharge Potential and Overall Status

Content. This section records whether the resident wants to return to the community, and whether there is a support person—usually a family member or friend—who is positive about the resident's discharge. It also records whether this nursing home stay is expected to be short term or of indefinite duration, and whether the resident has improved or declined overall in the past 90 days.

Clinical use. When discharge is desired or expected, the psychiatric evaluation should focus on any mental, behavioral, or social factors that might impede discharge or make a community placement unsuccessful. Mental and behavioral barriers to discharge are a strong indication for psychiatric consultation and implementation of a psychiatric care plan. Psychiatric interventions can promote residents' self-sufficiency and help them resolve conflicts with family caregivers. An emphasis on discharge potential can be useful to the psychiatrist in gaining the cooperation of residents, family members, and professionals of other disciplines.

Quarterly MDS Assessment

Residents receiving subacute care or rehabilitation under the Medicare skilled nursing facility benefit must have full MDS assessments on or about days 5, 14, 30, 60, and 90 of their nursing home stay. All other residents must have a full MDS annually and quarterly updates in between. The quarterly MDS comprises a subset of MDS items. Cognitive function, mood, and behavior items are included; items on pain and on psychosocial well-being are not.

Using the MDS in Psychiatry

Making Consultation More Efficient

At the resident's bedside, the MDS can focus attention on areas of abnormality. Areas normal on the MDS can be screened more briefly, especially if staff say that those areas have not changed significantly since the last MDS assessment. References to the MDS in the consultation report can facilitate communication with nursing facility staff.

When asking nursing staff to monitor a resident's response to a treatment, or to screen the resident periodically for side effects, the psychiatrist can draw many of the items to be monitored directly from the MDS. More generally, relating psychiatric diagnosis and treatment recommendations to the MDS and the RAPs leverages the staff's knowledge and increases their motivation. Staff know that surveyors will focus on QIs and on implementation of the RAPs. RAP protocols include those on mood, cognitive function, and behavioral problems. The psychiatrist who regularly consults to nursing facilities should be familiar with the RAP guidelines dealing with psychiatric issues.

Transferring Information to the Nursing Home From the Hospital or Clinic

When a nursing home receives timely, accurate, and sufficient information about a patient who has cognitive, behavioral, or mood problems, its staff can make an informed decision about admitting the patient. Patients who are inappropriate for a facility will be turned down, whereas those who fit the facility's capabilities especially well may be admitted sooner. When patients are admitted, their assignment to a particular unit, roommate, or primary nurse will be more likely to meet their needs. Initial care plans may be better and may be implemented sooner.

Because nursing homes must have staff familiar with the MDS, a partially completed MDS is a communication that will be understood. Because nursing home staff must complete an MDS on every newly admitted resident, a partially completed MDS can be a starting point for their own complete admission MDS.

Transferring Information to the Hospital or Clinic From the Nursing Home

When a nursing home resident is sent to a hospital or clinic, the clinicians receiving the resident can provide better care if they know the resident's baseline functioning and routines and are aware of any guardianship or advance medical directives. This information often is not transferred in emergency situations, in which the focus is on the acute problem. By sending a copy of the MDS along with the resident, the psychiatrist can provide answers to important questions about the resident's baseline, which can prevent over-treatment or under-treatment of acute problems. For example, knowing that a delirious patient had good cognitive functioning at baseline will prevent medical staff from denying the patient aggressive medical treatment on the assumption that the patient is irreversibly demented. Similarly, excessively vigorous treatment may be prevented if the staff know that a resident has poor baseline functioning and an advance directive limiting treatment.

The MDS will function best in this role if the clinicians receiving the patient understand how to read and interpret it. The psychiatrist, the primary care physician, or a nurse at the nursing home can attach a brief note to the front of the MDS that directs the reader to the scales most relevant to the situation at hand. Appendix C contains a sample of this type of referral note.

Monitoring Treatment Interventions

Most of the interventions suggested or prescribed by the psychiatrist in the nursing home are aimed at improving the resident's cognition, mood, or behavior or at eliminating side effects of psychotropic drugs. Secondary goals may include reducing the use of physical restraints or improving the resident's well-being, physical functioning, nutrition, and continence. Because these outcomes are reflected in MDS scales, the psychiatrist can monitor consequences of a nursing home resident's psychiatric treatment by having nursing home staff repeat selected MDS scales.

A comprehensive form for monitoring psychiatric treatment outcome in the nursing home would include the MDS scales for cognition, mood, behavior, well-being, restraints, physical ADLs, and continence; a disorder-specific scale such as the Hamilton Rating Scale for Depression; and a quantitative or semiquantitative rating that addresses the specific symptom of greatest concern. Examples of the latter include measuring body weight in a patient who was failing to thrive due to depression or rating the level of screaming in a patient for whom yelling for help was the most troublesome symptom.

The use of structured symptom ratings built around the MDS can increase the efficiency of the consultant's visits to the nursing home by reducing the time needed to elicit the resident's history and question the staff about effects of treatment. Also, keeping copies of such ratings in the office chart may help the psychiatrist comply with Medicare requirements for documenting the intensity and necessity of services provided.

Supporting and Documenting Psychotropic Drug Use

Nursing home regulations approve psychotropic drugs for the treatment of diagnosed mental illness or for the treatment of mental symptoms that significantly affect the resident's functioning and well-being. The MDS helps to establish diagnostic criteria and indicates when a resident's functions and well-being are impaired. A quarterly MDS repeated after apparently successful drug treatment can help establish that regulatory criteria for appropriate drug use were met. For example, if medication is used to treat a diagnosed mental illness, the psychiatrist can use the MDS to show that the drugs improved the mental symptoms without adverse effect on the resident's physical functioning or continence. If medication is used primarily to improve the resident's functioning or

well-being, the facility can use the MDS to show that the resident's functioning has improved. If the nursing home staff are reluctant to complete an extra quarterly MDS for this purpose, the psychiatrist can remind them that the quarterly MDS is to be completed ahead of schedule if the resident's clinical status has changed significantly.

Working With Families

Like nurses and regulators, family members may have reservations about the psychiatric treatment recommended for a nursing home resident. A commonly expressed fear is that medication will overly sedate a resident or make the resident "like a zombie." Using the framework of the MDS, the psychiatrist can explain that the treatment of psychiatric disorders and symptoms is intended to improve the resident's functioning and well-being, with a commitment to modify treatment if side effects occur. The psychiatrist can emphasize that mere control of specific symptoms is not sufficient, if it comes at the cost of diminished functioning (e.g., less time active, more impaired cognition, new-onset incontinence). The MDS is used as a tangible catalyst for a dialogue to promote collaboration and cooperation.

A related strategy concerns family involvement in the initial placement of a patient in a nursing home. The family can be given an MDS form during the nursing home search process and fill out those sections related to the patient's background, routine, legal status, mood, cognition, behavior, and continence. They can be encouraged to use the MDS as a tool in talking with nursing home staff about the patient's needs, ensuring that the staff know about the patient's baseline capabilities and preferred routine. This strategy can reduce the family's guilt by helping them become advocates for better, more individualized care (Morris and Lipsitz 1996).

References

Morris J, Lipsitz L (eds): Quality Care in the Nursing Home. St. Louis, MO, Mosby, 1996

Omnibus Budget Reconciliation Act: Public Law 100-203 (1987). Subtitle C, Nursing Home Reform. Washington, DC, U.S. General Printing Office, 1987

Useful Web Sites

www.hcfa.gov

This is the home page for the Health Care Financing Administration. Links will take the user to current information on the Medicare skilled nursing facility payment system and to results of the most recent surveys of each of the nation's Medicare- or Medicaid-certified nursing facilities.

www.aanac.org

This is the home page for the American Association of Nurse Assessment Coordinators. It has news of recent regulatory and payment policies, as well as convenient downloads of Health Care Financing Administration manuals and forms.

http://linear.chsra.wisc.edu

The University of Wisconsin Center for Health Systems Research and Analysis developed nursing facility Quality Indicators under a contract from the Health Care Financing Administration. Its Web site has detailed information about the Quality Indicators and other topics related to quality of care in nursing facilities.

Chapter 5

Introduction to OBRA-87 and Its Implications for Psychiatric Care

Each psychiatrist who participates in nursing home care needs to become familiar with the assessment and care provision requirements set forth in the Nursing Home Reform Act of 1987. The U.S. Congress commissioned a study by the Institute of Medicine in the mid-1980s to evaluate the quality of care in nursing homes (Institute of Medicine 1986). In response to this study, nursing home reform became a part of the Omnibus Reconciliation Act of 1987 (OBRA-87; Public Law 100-203). Congress mandated the development of a national resident assessment system for nursing facilities and set into motion admission and treatment guidelines that directly affect the quality of care of residents in nursing facilities. By July 1, 1995, the enforcement and penalty provisions regarding standards for drug administration, physical and somatic treatment of behavioral disorders, and other pertinent issues of resident rights went into effect and are part of the typical survey process of long-term care facilities (Medicare and Medicaid programs 1994).

Nursing home care is highly diverse. Caring for nursing facility residents is often complex and challenging because of the generally advanced age of residents, multiple illnesses, rehabilitative issues, psychosocial needs, and the frequency with which decisions need to be made by surrogates. Table 5–1 lists ten categories of high-risk care in the nursing home setting (Selma et al. 1994).

Assessment Provisions: Preadmission Screening and Resident Review

For psychiatrists who treat mental illness in nursing homes, the preadmission screening and resident review (PASRR) is an important component of OBRA legislation. This federal mandate requires an interdisciplinary PASRR evaluation prior to placement for patients who are requesting nursing home admission and who have symp-

Table 5–1. Categories of high-risk care in the nursing home setting

Treating symptoms, not causes

Treating conditions without sufficient assessment or reassessment

Deciding not to treat certain conditions without documenting justifications appropriately

Failing to follow up on test abnormalities

Failing to take action regarding an observed problem

Failing to recognize obvious complications or side effects

Using psychotropic medications without adequate evaluation, documentation, and reassessment

Editorializing in the chart

Failing to involve and communicate with families or surrogates

Providing care not reflected in the interdisciplinary care plan

toms or a diagnosis of mental illness, are receiving psychotropic drug treatment, or have experienced cognitive change. Serious mental illness includes schizophrenia; mood disorders; paranoia; panic or other severe anxiety disorders; somatoform disorders; personality disorders; other psychotic disorders; or other mental disorders that may lead to chronic disability (Medicare and Medicaid programs 1992). Patients who have a primary diagnosis of Alzheimer's disease or other dementia are excluded from the federal definition of serious mental illness and meet exception criteria.

The PASRR evaluation has two purposes: 1) to determine whether nursing home care is necessary for the patient based on physical and medical needs and 2) to determine whether specialty mental health services are required in order to care for the patient while he or she lives in the nursing home.

The PASRR evaluation includes a DSM-IV multiaxial diagnosis and mental health treatment recommendations. Recommendations may be made for specialized mental health services (i.e., professional mental health services) or other mental health services provided by the nursing home (e.g., psychosocial interventions such as group, environmental changes, and visitation). The OBRA team may ask a psychiatrist whose patient is planning to enter the nursing home for input with respect to the patient's psychiatric assessment, historical response to treatment, and ongoing treatment recommendations. The psychiatrist can provide valuable input to the OBRA team by advocating for the importance of ongoing mental health services and by making recommendations on the type and frequency of mental health intervention.

If a less restrictive environment would meet the patient's care needs adequately, the OBRA team will recommend alternative placement to the nursing home. If a patient residing in the nursing home no longer requires basic nursing care, the state must orchestrate a discharge to a less restrictive facility and must facilitate the patient's access to specialized mental health services.

For residents determined to have a mental illness, the PASRR evaluation is repeated annually and during times of significant mental status or behavioral change. This annual review describes the outcomes of treatment interventions over the past year and reassesses the resident's ongoing need for nursing home placement and specialized mental health services. A PASRR evaluation may also be initiated by nursing home staff or by a physician if a patient without a history of mental illness develops symptoms after nursing home admission.

Each nursing home is charged with carrying out the placement and treatment recommendations that result from the PASRR evaluation. Specialized mental health services must be provided by appropriately trained nursing home staff, the local community mental health board, or a private mental health professional within the community. Results of the PASRR assessment are provided to the referring individual, patient, and nursing home. Although criticized as being a variable database, PASRR evaluations are being assessed by some states as mechanisms to determine the extent of mental illness and service utilization in the nursing home setting.

Development of a positive working relationship with the OBRA team will allow the nursing home psychiatrist to gain additional helpful information about his or her patients. The PASRR evaluation contains data on the patient's functional status, current and previous medications, medical illness, and previous psychiatric treatments and response. The psychiatrist should review the PASRR data before the patient interview because the PASRR evaluation represents an independent source of patient information, in addition to nursing home staff input.

Assessment Provisions: The Resident Assessment Instrument

Assessment of patients' strengths, weaknesses, and problems has always been a key to providing psychiatric care in any setting. In long-term care, the Nursing Home Reform Act of 1987 mandated a national resident assessment system that includes a uniform set of items and definitions for assessing all residents (Public Law 100-203). In 1990, the Resident Assessment Instrument (RAI) was published as the foundation for assessing and delivering care. The RAI consists of a Minimum Data Set (MDS) and Resident Assessment Protocols (RAPs), common definitions and coding categories needed to perform a comprehensive assessment of a long-term care facility resident. Utilization Guidelines were provided by the Health Care Financing Administration (HCFA) in the form of the *Resident Assessment Instrument User's Manual*. The MDS was developed with a clinical focus, with the developers asking for each item in the document, "Is this something that clinicians need to know in order to provide care for a nursing home resident?" (Morris et al. 1990). The RAPs are "triggered" by MDS items and are intended to provide standardized decision frameworks, with guidelines for additional assessment of relevant resident attributes, risk factors, clinical history, and other factors. Thus, they assist with clinical decision making and help nursing home staff gather and analyze necessary information to develop an appropriate and individualized care plan. Additional benefits are to increase staff communication, increase the involvement of residents and their families in care planning and delivery, and improve documentation. Having applications outside the field of assessment as such but of far-reaching importance for reimbursement of clinical services provided to residents in long-term care facilities, the MDS is also the basis of the case-mix classification system (prospective payment system). This system is based on the "Resource Utilization Groups III, which is a mechanism for determining the level of resources necessary to care for an individual based upon his clinical characteristics as measured by the MDS" (Medicare and Medicaid 1997, p. 67174).

Because long-term nursing home care is so complex, a plan of care requires clinical competence, observation skills, and assessment expertise on the part of all disciplines. The RAI is designed to look at residents holistically with an emphasis on quality of life and quality of care (Morris et al. 1990). The nursing home team prepares an individualized comprehensive care plan by utilizing 1) the core set of screening, clinical, and functional status elements of the MDS and 2) the structured, problem-oriented frameworks of the RAPs. This care plan addresses each aspect of the resident's medical, nursing, rehabilitative, nutritional, psychosocial, and recreational life in the facility. The psychiatrist is often called in to evaluate a resident when the resident's medical, mental, functional, or psychosocial status has changed. The psychiatrist becomes an integral part of the assessment and care-planning process.

The *Resident Assessment Instrument User's Manual* gives specific details of the assessment process (Department of Health and Human Services 1995). The manual stresses four basic themes:

1. The resident is an individual with strengths, as a well as functional limitations and health problems.
2. Possible causes for each problem and guidance for further assessment, resolution, or interventions are presented in the RAPs.
3. An interdisciplinary approach to resident care is vital both in assessment and in development of a plan of care.
4. Good clinical practice requires solid, thorough assessment.

Figure 5–1 illustrates the RAI framework. Although the RAI assessment must occur at specific times according to federal regulations (Table 5–2),

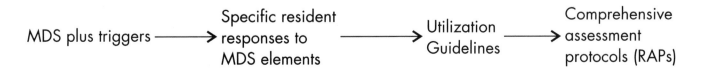

MDS plus triggers ⟶ Specific resident responses to MDS elements ⟶ Utilization Guidelines ⟶ Comprehensive assessment protocols (RAPs)

Figure 5–1. Resident Assessment Instrument (RAI) framework. MDS = Minimum Data Set; RAPs = Resident Assessment Protocols.

Table 5–2. Mandated time frames for Resident Assessment Instrument (RAI) assessment

Type of assessment	Time frame
Admission (initial) assessment	Must be complete by 14th day of resident's stay
Annual reassessment	Must be completed within 12 months of most recent full assessment
Significant change in status reassessment	Must be completed by the end of 14th calendar day following determination of significant change
Quarterly assessment	Set of MDS items, mandated by state (containing minimal HCFA subset), must be completed at least every 3 months

Note. MDS = Minimum Data Set; HCFA = Health Care Financing Administration.

a facility's obligation to meet residents' needs through ongoing assessment is not confined to the mandated time frame. From a psychiatric standpoint, significant changes include changes in the resident's decision making or cognitive status, emergence of sad or anxious mood patterns, increase in the number of behavioral symptoms, emergence of unplanned weight loss, or the initial need of physical restraints.

The MDS contains information about the resident's mental health history (see Chapter 4). As with the PASRR evaluation, the MDS defines a mental health condition if a resident has a documented history of schizophrenia; mood disorders; paranoia; panic or other severe anxiety disorder; somatoform disorders; personality disorders; other psychiatric disorders; or another mental disorder that may lead to chronic disability. A primary diagnosis of dementia is an exception criterion.

One of the following qualifications also must be met:

- The disorder resulted in functional limitations in major life activities within the past 3–6 months.
- The treatment history indicates that the resident has had psychiatric care more intensive

than outpatient care more than once in past 2 years *or* received formal support services in order to maintain functioning at home.

Residents are also screened for mental retardation and developmental disabilities. This does not mean that residents with these conditions cannot reside in a long-term care facility, but it enables the nursing home to plan and provide appropriate care for them.

The social history provides background information about the resident's lifestyle, education, work, and use of substances. The functional assessment portion of the MDS examines cognitive patterns, including cognitive skills for decision making and indicators for delirium; communication and hearing patterns; mood and behavior patterns; pain symptoms; and medication use, particularly psychotropic medications.

After the MDS has been completed, the resident's *triggers* are determined. If specific items or a combination of items point to a problem or potential problem, an RAP is used to determine a strategy for further assessment and solution. For example, a delirium protocol would be triggered if a resident exhibited easy distractibility; periods of altered perception or awareness; disorganized speech; restlessness; lethargy; variability of cognition over the day; or deterioration of cognitive status, mood, or behaviors. An RAP is then completed to determine if the problem has a reversible cause. The RAP outlines diagnoses as well as conditions that could contribute to the symptoms, including medications, psychosocial reasons, and sensory impairments. The RAP would guide the OBRA team in planning care that would correct reversible causes of symptoms and in planning somatic or behavioral interventions to assist the resident during this time.

RAPS are available to address changes in cognition, mood, and behavior. The psychiatrist must be aware of the key questions the OBRA team must answer in order to complete RAPs and care plans. The psychiatrist 's assessment of the resident may play an important part in the comprehensive assessment and treatment plan, particularly when questions exist about the resident's mental impairment due to delirium, the presence of an affective disorder, or the resident's psychosocial adjustment to placement or change in functional status. Within this section of the RAI is the mandate that a comprehensive care plan be developed in conjunction with the OBRA team and the resident or surrogate to develop "quantifiable objectives for the highest level of functioning the resident may be expected to attain." The staff will use documentation of the mental status examination, differential diagnoses, concomitant medical illnesses, and psychiatric care planning to plan care for the resident.

advise that the resident should receive appropriate treatment and services to correct the assessed problem. These assessments include thorough evaluation of clinical presentation, communication losses, physical or social isolation, sleep-wake cycle abnormalities, spiritual or cultural needs, and potential for violence or any stereotyped responses to any stressor. The psychiatrist's role will be to evaluate from a biopsychosocial approach the resident's behavioral problems, including physical symptoms, medications, psychiatric disorders, dementia, social problems, and developmental dilemmas.

Resident Rights Provisions

OBRA-87 regulations also require familiarity with basic resident rights. These include

> Ensur[ing] that the resident is informed of his/her health status including functional status, medical care, nursing care, nutritional status, rehabilitation potential, activities potential, health status, psychosocial status, and sensory/physical impairments. (Department of Health and Human Services 1995)

Also key to resident rights is that the resident has the right to refuse treatment, to refuse to participate in "experimental research," and to participate to the best of his or her abilities in the formulation of advance directives. The fact that the resident has a right to refuse treatment in no way absolves the facility and caregivers from providing care so that the resident is able to achieve his or her highest potential.

The resident also has a right to be free of restraints, both physical and chemical. A chemical restraint is defined by the regulations as a psychopharmacologic drug used for discipline or for staff convenience to address behavioral symptoms and not required to treat medical symptoms. The regulations also describe "unnecessary drugs," which are defined later in this chapter.

For a resident who shows mental or psychosocial adjustment difficulty, regulations

Treatment Provisions

If a resident is receiving or is deemed to require psychotropic medications, the guidelines advise that although psychopharmacologic drugs can be "therapeutic and enabling" for residents with mental illness, psychotropic medications should not be used solely or excessively to address certain behavioral symptoms. The implementation of the regulations has had a significant effect on the prescribing habits in nursing homes. A study in Minnesota nursing homes reported that 23% of nursing home residents were administered antipsychotic drugs before the guidelines were implemented. By 1990–1991, after the guidelines were in effect, this percentage had declined to 15% (Garrard et al. 1995). A Tennessee study noted a 26.7% reduction of antipsychotic drug use after the date on which the guidelines were announced (Shorr et al. 1994). This study showed not only a reduction in new users but also a reduction of long-term use of antipsychotic drugs. A collaborative study from New York and Philadelphia investigated the relationship between physical restraint reduction and the use of psychoactive drugs in the wake of OBRA-87 (Siegler 1997). Interventions to reduce physical restraints in nursing homes did not lead to an increase in psychoactive drug use. This study also found that when a structured educational program was used, antipsychotic use declined dramatically.

The regulations state that nursing home residents must be free from unnecessary drugs, which are defined as

- Drugs used in excessive dosages (as listed below unless there is documentation that higher dosages are required to improve the resident's function)
- Drugs used in excessive duration (daily use for greater than 4 months unless a gradual dosage reduction was unsuccessful)
- Drugs prescribed without adequate monitoring of side effects
- Drugs prescribed without adequate indications for use
- Drug continued in the presence of adverse consequences
- Any combination of the above

Descriptions of Individual Drug Classes

Benzodiazepines

The guidelines recommend that long-acting benzodiazepines be avoided unless an attempt to use a short-acting drug has failed. These regulations are not enforced in the following situations:

- If the resident is given diazepam for neuromuscular syndromes such as cerebral palsy, tardive dyskinesia, or seizure disorder
- If long-acting benzodiazepines are used to withdraw residents from short-acting drugs
- If clonazepam is used to treat bipolar disorder, nocturnal myoclonus, or seizure disorder

Table 5–3 outlines the prescribing recommendations for benzodiazepines.

Recommended indications for benzodiazepines include generalized anxiety disorder, panic disorder, organic mental syndromes that are persistent and not preventable and that cause distress or dysfunction, and symptomatic anxiety in residents with another diagnosed psychiatric disorder (e.g., depression, adjustment disorder).

The recommended duration for daily use of long-acting benzodiazepines is less than 4 months. After this period, dosage reduction

Table 5–3.   Maximum recommended total daily doses of benzodiazepines

Drug	Daily oral dosage[a] (mg)
Alprazolam	0.75
Chlorazepate	15
Chlordiazepoxide	20
Diazepam	5
Estazolam	0.5
Flurazepam	15
Halazepam	40
Lorazepam	2
Oxazepam	30
Quazepam	7.5

[a]Unless a higher dose is documented for improvement in functional status.

should be attempted. Dosage reduction and elimination should be tried at least twice a year for short-acting benzodiazepines.

Hypnotics

Clinicians should remember that diminished nighttime sleep is not necessarily pathologic and that other possible causes of sleep-wake disturbance (e.g., pain, depression, environmental causes, caffeine or other drugs) should be ruled out before hypnotics are prescribed. Table 5–4 outlines the prescribing recommendations for hypnotics.

Table 5–4.   Recommended dosages of hypnotics

Drug[a]	Daily oral dosage (mg)
Alprazolam	0.25
Choral hydrate	500
Diphenhydramine	25
Estazolam	0.5
Hydroxyzine	50
Lorazepam	1
Oxazepam	15
Temazepam	7.5
Triazolam	0.125
Zolpidem	5

[a]Diphenhydramine, hydroxyzine, and choral hydrate are listed but are not recommended by the regulations.

The patient should not take a hypnotic for more than 10 consecutive days. Gradual dosage reduction should be attempted at least three times within a 6-month period before the clinician can conclude that a gradual dosage reduction is clinically contraindicated.

The following sleep-inducing drugs should not be given to any nursing home resident:

- Amobarbital
- Amobarbital-secobarbital combination
- Barbiturates with other drugs
- Butabarbital
- Ethchlorvynol
- Glutethimide
- Meprobamate
- Methyprylon
- Paraldehyde
- Pentobarbital
- Phenobarbital (except if used for seizure control)
- Secobarbital

A newly admitted resident should be given a period of adjustment before gradual withdrawal of any of these drugs. No rapid withdrawal should be encouraged.

Antipsychotics

Table 5–5 outlines the prescribing recommendations for antipsychotics.

Antipsychotics should not be prescribed unless the nursing home resident is being treated for one of the following disorders:

- Schizophrenia
- Schizoaffective disorder
- Delusional disorder
- Psychotic mood disorders (including bipolar disorder with psychotic features, acute psychotic reaction, brief psychotic reaction, schizophreniform disorder, atypical psychosis)
- Tourette's syndrome, Huntington's disease, short-term treatment of specific disorders—hiccups, nausea, vomiting, itching

For treatment of organic mental syndrome with antipsychotic drugs, the following symptoms must exist:

- Psychotic symptoms and/or agitated behaviors that are persistent or not caused by reversible etiologies
- Symptoms not responsive to behavioral interventions
- Behaviors causing a danger to the resident or others
- Symptoms that persistently impair functional capacity (e.g., constant yelling, screaming, or repetitive behaviors)

Table 5–5. Maximum recommended daily dosages of antipsychotics

Drug	Daily oral dosage for residents with "organic mental syndromes"[a,b] (mg)
Acetophenazine	20
Chlorpromazine	75
Chlorprothixene	75
Clozapine	50
Fluphenazine	4
Haloperidol	4
Loxapine	10
Mesoridazine	25
Molindone	10
Perphenazine	8
Prochlorperazine[c]	10
Promazine	150
Risperidone	2
Thioridazine	75
Thiothixene	7
Trifluoperazine	8
Triflupromazine	20

[a]The term *organic mental syndrome* is considered obsolete. It is included here only because of existing OBRA regulatory language.
[b]Antipsychotic drugs should not be used in excess of these daily dosages unless higher dosages are necessary to maintain or improve the resident's functional status.
[c]The dosage of prochlorperazine may be exceeded for short-term (7-day) treatment of nausea and vomiting. Residents who have cancer with nausea and vomiting may use it for longer periods of time at higher doses.

The guidelines deem antipsychotic drugs unnecessary under the following conditions:

- If given in higher than advised dosages without adequate documentation
- If given without due regard to the diagnosis
- If adequate monitoring for adverse effects such as tardive dyskinesia, hypotension, cognitive or behavioral impairment, akathisia, and parkinsonism is not documented
- If gradual reduction is not attempted

Antipsychotics should not be used if one or more of the following symptoms is the only indication:

- Agitated behaviors that do not represent a danger to self or others
- Anxiety
- Depression
- Fidgeting
- Impaired memory
- Indifference to surroundings
- Insomnia
- Lack of cooperation
- Nervousness
- Poor self-care
- Restlessness
- Unsociability
- Wandering

The guidelines state that "Residents who use antipsychotic drugs must receive gradual dose reductions and behavioral interventions, unless clinically contraindicated, in an effort to discontinue these drugs." Even though the guidelines do not give a specific time frame, evaluation at least quarterly is necessary.

Antidepressants

Antidepressants are underutilized in nursing home care and have not been subjected to the same criterion for gradual dosage reduction applied to anxiolytics (i.e., benzodiazepines), hypnotics, and antipsychotics. According to the guidelines, when prescribing antipsychotics, the psychiatrist must do the following:

- Assess the patient's need for medication.
- Use medication dosages appropriate for a geriatric population or document the reasons for higher dosages.
- Monitor effects (noting any untoward side effects).
- Use the least anticholinergic drugs available.

Required Documentation

When prescribing *any* psychotherapeutic medication in a nursing home setting, the psychiatrist must ensure that

- A medical or psychiatric consultation or evaluation confirms the necessity of the drug regimen (including the duration of the drug use, attempts at dosage reduction, and explanation of any dosages that exceed guideline recommendations).
- In the case of antipsychotics, the diagnosis is documented, the symptoms described, and behavioral interventions considered before or in conjunction with the somatic treatment.
- The risks and benefits of psychotherapeutic medication are spelled out to the resident or surrogate and this process is documented.
- The positive and negative effects of medication are monitored and documented.
- Gradual dosage reduction attempts or reduction failures are documented.
- Subjective and objective measures of the resident's functioning are documented during the medication regimen.
- In the face of a resident's functional or medical deterioration while on psychotherapeutic medication, a thorough medical evaluation is completed and the medication regimen reconsidered.

For more information, see The OBRA '87 Enforcement Rule: Implications for Attending Physicians and Medical Directors. Columbia, MD,

American Medical Directors Association, 1995. Available from the American Medical Directors Association, 10480 Little Patuxent Parkway, Suite 760, Columbia, MD 21044.

Questions concerning the RAI, version 2.0, can be referred to the following address: MDS Coordinator, Center on Long Term Care, Health Standards and Quality Bureau, Health Care Financing Administration, 7500 Security Boulevard, Baltimore, MD 21244-1850.

References

Department of Health and Human Services: State Operations Manual: Provider Certification (Transmittal #272). Baltimore, MD, Health Care Financing Administration, 1995

Garrard J, Chen V, Dowd B: The impact of the 1987 federal regulations on the use of psychotropic drugs in Minnesota nursing homes. Am J Public Health 85:771–776, 1995

Institute of Medicine: Improving Quality of Care in Nursing Homes. Washington, DC, National Academy Press, 1986

Medicare and Medicaid programs; preadmission screening and annual resident review—HCFA. Federal Register 57(230):56450–56514, November 30, 1992

Medicare and Medicaid programs; survey certification and enforcement of skilled nursing facilities and nursing facilities—HCFA; final rule. Federal Register 59(217):56116–56252, November 10, 1994

Medicare and Medicaid; resident assessment in long term care facilities—HCFA. Federal Register 62(246):67174–67213, December 12, 1997

Morris JN, Hawes C, Fries BE, et al: Designing the national resident assessment instrument for nursing homes. Gerontologist 30:292–303, 1990

Omnibus Budget Reconciliation Act: Public Law 100-203 (1987). Subtitle C, Nursing Home Reform. Washington, DC, U.S. Government Printing Office, 1987

Selma TP, Palla K, Poddig B, et al: Effect of the Omnibus Reconciliation Act 1987 on antipsychotic prescribing in nursing home residents. J Am Geriatr Soc 42:648–652, 1994

Shorr RI, Fought RL, Ray WA: Changes in antipsychotic drug use in nursing homes during implementation of the OBRA-87 regulations. JAMA 271:358–362, 1994

Siegler EL, Capezuti E, Maislin G, et al: Effects of a restraint reduction intervention and OBRA'87 regulations on psychoactive drug use in nursing homes. J Am Geriatr Soc 45:791–796, 1997

→

Section 3

Financial Aspects

Chapter 6

Documentation, Reimbursement, and Coding

Documentation

Medicare generally requires that services rendered to a patient must be reasonable and necessary for the diagnosis and active treatment of the patient's illness. Medicare will consistently deny reimbursement for services that do not meet their criteria of medical necessity, regardless of the site of service (e.g., hospital, nursing home, physician's office).

Services must be directed toward alleviation of impairments that precipitated the consultation or that necessitate continued intervention. They must enhance the patient's coping abilities, and they must be individualized to address the patient's specific needs.

The Health Care Financing Administration (HCFA) vests with local Medicare carriers considerable flexibility in implementing payment rules and review standards. Given recent enforcement activities in the area of mental illness treatment, it is of increasing importance for the psychiatrist to be certain of the technical accuracy of claims and to document all claims thoroughly. When serious questions arise, oral statements from carrier claims representatives should not be accepted as the carrier's final word. When in doubt, the psychiatrist should make every effort to obtain from the carrier written policy guidance.

At the inpatient and partial hospitalization level and in nursing homes, more patient charts are being reviewed by third-party carriers than ever before. Claims are being rejected for which information in the patient's chart does not meet criteria for severity of illness and intensity of service screening used by local Medicare carriers and peer-review organizations. Services provided to patients whose need for or ability to benefit from active psychiatric treatment may be questioned will almost certainly be denied.

When asked to see a patient, the psychiatrist should ensure that the consultation order has been written by the patient's attending physician or the facility's medical director and that it includes clear documentation of the reason the consultation has been requested. The psychiatrist should not initiate treatment unless a specific request to do so is made.

Documentation is absolutely essential to getting paid. When consulting in a nursing home, the psychiatrist should provide the same level of comprehensive documentation that is required in a hospital setting. The initial note, a brief notation of the findings and recommendations of an initial psychiatric evaluation or consultation, should include the reason or justification for consultation, results of a brief mental status examination, a list of current medications and concomitant medical problems, and a preliminary treatment plan outlining short-term and long-term goals.

A comprehensive psychiatric evaluation should be completed and recorded in the patient's chart in a timely manner. If the patient has been evaluated previously, an updated evaluation will do. The evaluation should clearly show the patient's current mental status and the changes that have necessitated the psychiatric consultation or follow-up.

> *Each patient who requires active treatment must have an individualized treatment plan.*

The master treatment plan is a detailed outline of a work in progress and should include the following information:

- Identifying data
- 5-Axis diagnosis
- Strengths and liabilities
- Reason for the consultation
- Presenting problem(s)
- Long-term and short-term goals
- Patient objectives
- Multidisciplinary interventions and goals
- Criteria for discontinuation of treatment

The psychiatrist should review the treatment plan at regular intervals to evaluate the patient's progress toward the outlined goals and objectives. Revisions and modifications to the treatment plan should be made when indicated.

At each visit, the psychiatrist should write a progress note. The note should contain the following elements: a brief observation of the patient's mental status, contents of the individual session, the intervention recommended or ordered, the patient's response to treatment, and the patient's progress or lack of progress toward goals.

If after a reasonable trial, the patient has not made progress toward the desired goals and objectives, then another level of care may be indicated.

> *The patient's chart must tell a story. There must be a clear picture of 1) the patient's movement from one level of care to another, 2) the patient's progress within the treatment program, 3) the changes made if the patient failed to respond as expected, 4) the effect of those changes on the patient, and 5) plans for the patient's eventual discharge from the active treatment plan.*

Reimbursement

The HCFA is giving increasing scrutiny to the shifting, from in-house to outside providers, of psychosocial and behavioral health services that nursing homes are expected to provide. Some facilities have met this responsibility by contracting directly with psychiatrists to provide care for their patients. Under this arrangement the psychiatrist would receive compensation directly from the nursing home and would not seek reimbursement from either the patient or Medicare Part B. Although rare, this arrangement most nearly meets some Medicare carrier's most stringent interpretation.

Many facilities provide some level of in-house assessment to meet the patient's psychosocial needs. Nursing and social services staff work closely with the attending physician to develop and carry out treatment plans with the primary goals of alleviating symptoms and modifying behavior. A psychiatrist is consulted only after documented and unsuccessful attempts to manage and improve the patient's condition. In this case the psychiatrist seeks reimbursement under Part B but provides only very specific and limited treatment and orders behavior-modifying treatment modalities to be carried out by the facility's staff.

A few facilities have attempted to shift all responsibility for delivery of psychosocial services to outside providers. This is clearly not appropriate under current HCFA guidelines.

A great deal of discussion is going on about the degree of medical and psychiatric care that nursing homes can and should provide. As the age and medical complexity of nursing home residents escalates, there is increasing concern that patients should be able to receive from qualified providers care that is appropriate for their condition. The HCFA's goal is not to deny treatment to patients in nursing homes but to ensure that the care provided is appropriate and medically necessary and that reimbursement is obtained from the proper source.

This goal has put some psychiatrists in the position of having their claims for conscientiously provided services denied. An unscrupulous few of these outside providers have been charged with overstating the intensity of the service provided or with delivery of medically unnecessary or outright fraudulent services to "captive" patients in long-term care settings.

Proper documentation should not be taken lightly. It is absolutely essential in order to receive reimbursement for the services rendered. The provider should expect that 100% of his or her charts will be reviewed, and he or she should prepare for that event.

> *Take the time to develop a systematic method of proper documentation. It will soon become second nature.*

Other Mental Health Providers and "Incident to . . . " Services

In a common practice model the psychiatrist or nurse practitioner evaluates and medically manages patients' mental health problems, and a social worker, nurse practitioner, or psychologist provides individual, group, or family therapy "incident to" the physician's care for patients requiring the services. Although this model is usually acceptable in the physician's office, this same "incident to . . . " privilege does not extend to the hospital and nursing home.

The Balanced Budget Act of 1997 provides for prospective payment and consolidated billing of the package of services provided to nursing home residents covered by Medicare Part A. Although physicians, nurse practitioners, advanced practice nurse clinicians, and clinical psychologists are excluded from this bundled group of services, licensed clinical social workers (LCSWs) are not. Therefore, therapies provided by an LCSW are considered part of the package of services provided by the facility. As such, the services of an LCSW or any other provider not specifically excluded, cannot be considered "incident to" the physician's care. The consolidated billing requirement currently does not extend to those nursing home residents whose stay is not covered by

Medicare Part A, and an LCSW may continue to bill Medicare Part B for therapies provided to patients; however, it is expected that the consolidated billing requirement will be extended to include therapies provided to all nursing home residents by July 2000.

> *It is critical to understand your local Medicare carrier's policy on "incident to . . ." services before having other clinicians deliver services. Supervision and credentialing requirements may vary greatly.*

Coding

In 1997, new Health Care Financing Administration Common Procedural Coding System (HCPCS) Level II psychotherapy codes were introduced, which again recognized ongoing medical evaluation and management as a separate and distinct part of the overall treatment. The HCPCS Level II psychotherapy codes were incorporated fully into Current Procedural Terminology (CPT) codes in 1998. In 1997 Medicare providers could not use the psychotherapy codes listed in CPT.

Separate psychotherapy codes are now established for both office and inpatient settings. "Office or Other Outpatient" codes are used in physicians' offices, community mental health centers, hospital outpatient clinics, emergency rooms, and observation programs. They should also be used in structured outpatient programs other than partial hospitalization and in domiciliary or rest homes, custodial care settings, and home care settings. "Inpatient" codes are used in inpatient programs of general or psychiatric hospitals, partial hospitalization programs, residential treatment centers, and nursing homes.

The codes also make greater distinction between insight-oriented, behavior-modifying, or supportive psychotherapy and interactive psychotherapy:

- Insight-oriented psychotherapy alleviates symptoms.

- Behavior-modifying psychotherapy develops adapted behaviors.
- Supportive psychotherapy encourages personal growth.
- Interactive psychotherapy uses interactive techniques as a mechanism of nonverbal communication.

The interactive psychotherapy code was developed primarily to describe play therapy with children, but millions of units of interactive psychotherapy have been billed to Medicare! The code pays slightly more than insight-oriented psychotherapy. Psychiatrists may use the code if they believe it is appropriate, but they must be prepared to defend their position and to document it.

The new codes now differentiate psychotherapy furnished *without* medical management services from psychotherapy furnished *with* medical management services. By eliminating the word "medical" from "medical psychotherapy" and the phrase "by a physician," it is made clear that the use of codes to report psychotherapy without medical evaluation and management services is not re-

stricted to physicians and will be open to clinical psychologists and clinical social workers (Medicare program 1996). Medical evaluation and management services can be provided only by physicians, nurse practitioners, or clinical nurse specialists.

CPT specifies that only face-to-face time can be considered in selecting the proper code; other adjunctive activities associated with the psychotherapy session are not to be considered for coding purposes. Thus 20 minutes of psychotherapy plus 20 minutes of chart review at the nursing station equals 20 minutes of face-to-face psychotherapy. Similarly, when providing psychotherapy with medical evaluation and management services, the psychiatrist should consider only the face-to-face time spent in psychotherapy when selecting the proper code. Thus 20 minutes of psychotherapy plus 20 minutes of face-to-face medication review and instruction equals 20 minutes of psychotherapy with evaluation and management. Table 6–1 summarizes the new codes, which took effect January 1, 1998.

If less than 20 minutes of psychotherapy is provided along with drug management, the code for

Table 6–1. Current Procedural Terminology (CPT) codes, effective January 1, 1998

Place of service	Face-to-face time in psychotherapy	Psychotherapy only[a]	Psychotherapy with medical evaluation or management
Insight-oriented psychotherapy, behavior modification, and supportive psychotherapy			
Office or other outpatient setting	20–30 min	90804	90805
	45–50 min	90806	90807
	75–80 min	90808	90809
Inpatient, PHP, or residential care setting	20–30 min	90816	90817
	45–50 min	90818	90819
	75–80 min	90821	90822
Interactive psychotherapy			
Office or other outpatient setting	20–30 min	90810	90811
	45–50 min	90812	90813
	75–80 min	90814	90815
Inpatient, PHP, or residential care setting	20–30 min	90823	90824
	45–50 min	90826	90827
	75–80 min	90828	90829

[a]The shaded codes are restricted codes. Although payment for these services is available, Medicare carriers usually require that a written report be submitted with the claim.
Source. American Medical Association 1999.

psychopharmacologic management (90862) may be most appropriate. Some psychiatric procedure codes are designated as restricted. These are generally codes whose medical appropriateness or necessity may be difficult to determine without additional information or those codes used more frequently than projected and, therefore, raising questions of inappropriate utilization. Family psychotherapy, whether without the patient present (CPT code 90846) or with (CPT code 90847), remains a billable service; however, a written report of the service, substantiating its medical necessity, should be submitted with the claim in order to facilitate Medicare payment.

The HCFA has extended these same restrictions to codes 90816, 90818, 90821, 90823, 90826, and 90828 (psychotherapy provided without medical management in inpatient, partial hospitalization, or residential care settings; see shaded codes in Table 6–1) (Medicare Bulletin TN 96-12). When medical evaluation and management services are provided without psychotherapy, the appropriate nursing facility services evaluation and management (E/M) code should be used for subsequent care (99311–99313). Time is not considered a major factor in selecting the appropriate code; however, if more than half of the face-to-face time is spent in counseling the patient, then a code based on time alone may be used.

Consultation E/M codes are also site specific. The inpatient consultation codes (99251–99255) should also be used for residents of nursing facilities. However, codes 99241–99245, designated for office or other outpatient setting, should be used for those patients in domiciliary or custodial care settings.

> *Despite instructions in CPT, if asked to initiate recommended treatment, the consulting psychiatrist may not use the consultation code for the first patient encounter but should use the appropriate psychotherapy or E/M code for subsequent visits. This 1999 HCFA variance has been the subject of great outcry. Psychiatrists should consult their local Medicare carrier for exact interpretation of current policy.*

New E/M documentation guidelines were developed by the HCFA and the American Medical Association in 1997. These guidelines include detailed organ system–specific examination and documentation requirements for psychiatry. Because of widespread protests that the documentation requirements are in excess of those associated with clinically appropriate medical record–keeping practices, the HCFA has delayed their full implementation indefinitely. Medicare carriers have been directed to use both the 1995 and 1997 E/M guidelines, whichever is more advantageous to the physician.

Like the consultation and E/M codes, the new psychiatric codes are site specific. Great care should be taken to ensure that Medicare claims are coded properly for the place of service. A facility may provide many levels of residential and nursing care within its confines. The psychiatrist should ascertain the level of care the patient is receiving and select the correct code.

If physician services are rendered to a patient in a nursing facility, the place of service code should be 31 (skilled nursing facility), 32 (nursing facility), or 33 (custodial care facility), depending on the designated care level of the patient. Thus for a patient meeting the criteria for skilled care under Medicare or Medicaid the psychiatrist should use place of service code 31, whereas for a patient in the same skilled nursing facility who did not meet Medicare criteria for skilled care (or required only an intermediate level of care or intermediate care facility [ICF]) the psychiatrist should use place of service code 32. For services provided to residents of assisted living facilities, rest homes, or board and care homes, the psychiatrist should use code 33.

> *Contrary to popular belief, the 62.5% outpatient psychiatric limitation is not linked to the procedure code but to the diagnostic code and the place of service. All places of service other than regular admission to a hospital inpatient unit are considered outpatient for Medicare reimbursement purposes.*

Although some Medicare carriers have been slower to adopt this regulation than others, HCFA policy states that effective January 1, 1992, the 62.5% outpatient psychiatric limitation applies to most services for which the primary diagnosis is a mental disorder (i.e., ICD-9-CM diagnosis codes 290–319). Exceptions are made for initial psychiatric evaluations, initial consultations, psychiatric diagnostic procedures (CPT codes 90801–90802 and 96100–96117), and HCPCS M0064 (brief office visit for monitoring or changing drug prescriptions) (Medicare Bulletin, TN GR 92-5).

For example, If the Medicare *approved* charge for an outpatient psychiatric service is $100, Medicare will limit the charge to 62.5% of the approved amount, or $62.50. This becomes the *allowed* charge on which Medicare calculates its payment. Medicare pays 80% of the *allowed* amount, or $50. The patient or his or her supplemental insurer is responsible for the difference between the Medicare payment and the *approved* amount. This is calculated at 20% of the allowed charge ($12.50) plus the 37.5% outpatient psychiatric reduction ($37.50) for total of $50.)

> *Despite using the inpatient psychotherapy codes, the psychiatrist will receive Medicare reimbursement at the outpatient rate for all subsequent care provided to nursing home patients.*

A frequent misperception is that the 37.5% outpatient psychiatric reduction must be written off. In fact, a physician must make every reasonable effort to collect the full approved charge, even though Medicare pays an effective rate of only 50% of that amount (80% of 62.5% of the approved charge). The only exceptions to this are patients with dual Medicare-Medicaid eligibility or those participating in Medicare health maintenance organizations (HMOs). Most Medicaid programs pay less than the full coinsurance amount and require the balance to be adjusted; an HMO will have its own cost-sharing requirements.

> *A provider must make every reasonable effort to collect the full approved charge for outpatient psychiatric services, even though Medicare pays an effective rate of only 50% of that amount.*

References

American Medical Association CPT Editorial Advisory Board: CPT '99. Chicago, IL, American Medical Association, 1999, p 380

Medicare program; revisions to payment policies and five-year review of and adjustments to the relative value units under the physician fee schedule for calendar year 1997—HCFA. Federal Register 61(227):59490–59716, November 22, 1996

Medicare Bulletin, TN GR 92-5:9

Medicare Bulletin Special Release, TN 96-12:2–4, 33–35

Chapter 7

Contracting With Nursing Homes

The Psychiatrist as Medical Director

In the 1970s it became mandatory for nursing homes that provided skilled care to have a medical director. Before that time, nursing home medical care often was provided by semiretired physicians who focused almost exclusively on nursing home practice. Often one or two such physicians would care for all the patients in a nursing facility. Oversight and coordination of the quality of care was provided, if it occurred at all, by the nursing staff. The U.S. Congress subsequently mandated that skilled care facilities employ medical directors and even defined many of their responsibilities.

The basic functions of a medical director are defined by statute and regulation. Generally, these functions include oversight of all medical care provided in the facility. This means credentialing attending physicians, ensuring timeliness of visits, securing necessary consulting services (including psychiatric), and occasionally intervening in communication problems that arise between attending physicians and nursing staff. The medical director also serves on vital facility committees, such as infection control, ethics, safety, admissions, and other professional advisory committees.

The medical director does not necessarily have direct responsibility for the patients, something for which few psychiatrists would be qualified. Nevertheless, in many nursing homes, the medical director's position remains an outgrowth of the preexisting system of an attending physician devoting much of his or her practice life to the care of the residents. As in the past, such an individual may have retired from other clinical practice. He or she fulfills the necessary medical director functions while taking care of a large number of patients in the home.

In recent decades some nursing homes have had a different role for the medical director. These facilities may use a staff model similar to that of most hospitals. There the medical director has much more of a care oversight function. A number of physicians from the community may provide care, including physicians employed by the home (e.g., a psychiatrist, a subacute care director). In such a setting a psychiatrist may be eminently qualified, possibly even the best qualified physician, to fill the role of medical director.

The requirements of the job include interpersonal functions that are natural for psychiatrists. For example, the job includes making telephone contact with attending physicians regarding mandatory patient visits and documentation, listening to and assessing nursing staff concerns regarding care issues, and helping to decide whether a troublesome resident's moods and behaviors require psychiatric evaluation (and sometimes providing that evaluation personally). Vital to success in this role is relationship building with administration and senior members of the nursing staff and other departments, an area in which psychiatrists are often especially skilled.

Although some nursing facilities remain wedded to the practice of having the medical director obtain whatever reimbursement he or she can by billing residents for direct clinical services, an increasing number of facilities pay a salary to the medical director. The facility may be able to recover a portion of this expense in its Medicaid fee basis. This is a far preferable method of reimbursement, especially for psychiatrists who serve as medical directors. The functions that psychiatrists can best perform as medical directors are precisely those for which no direct reimbursement is possible. A salary permits the medical director to become a vital and valued member of or consultant to the management team. Although not every facility will recognize this, in the long run the psychiatrist's consultative and interpersonal skills are far more useful than is his or her sole provision of individual psychiatric care. This can be an extremely fulfilling type of employment, often part time, which can greatly enrich the career of a geriatric or general psychiatrist.

Function of the Contract

The contract is an important tool that enables the psychiatrist to develop a long-lasting, trusting relationship with the administrative staff of a long-term care facility. The piece of paper is not as important as the mutual trust and confidence that is built between the two parties. The nursing home administrator and director of nurses want assurance that the consulting psychiatrist will be available to meet in a dependable manner the psychiatric needs of the facility's residents and staff, and the psychiatrist wants assurance that the nursing home will be a long-term source of referrals for his or her practice. The contract becomes a tangible solution for these needs.

We have often thought of the nursing home itself as being the real patient in need of care. It is estimated that 51%–94% of all nursing home residents will meet the criteria for a psychiatric illness, ranging from dementia, to acute depression, to psychoses and schizophrenia, as may be observed in former patients of state hospitals (Tariot et al. 1993). Often the nursing home staff is poorly trained and ill prepared to manage these prob-

lems. The nursing home administrator, director of nurses, and nursing staff may be uneasy about managing the problems of psychiatric patients. It is the job of the consulting psychiatrist and his or her staff to treat this anxiety. The written contract is the first step in this process. The contract should clearly address the fears of the nursing home staff and administration, for example, by answering the following questions:

- Will the consulting psychiatrist be available for emergencies 24 hours per day?
- How long will it take to reach the consulting psychiatrist in an emergency?
- Will the consulting psychiatrist follow up with patients after the initial evaluation?
- Will the consulting psychiatrist be able to hospitalize patients when necessary?
- Will the consulting psychiatrist conform to Omnibus Reconciliation Act of 1987 (OBRA-87) requirements for psychotropic medication?
- Will the consulting psychiatrist make rounds on a frequent and regular schedule?

Signing a contract to deliver good service is the start of a potentially rewarding and lucrative relationship with a long-term care facility. Of course, the psychiatrist must follow through on the terms of the contract and provide timely and reliable service to the nursing home in order to be successful.

Contract Format

The owners and administrators of long-term care facilities are business people. They know little about clinical medicine. The psychiatrist is attempting to form a business relationship with the nursing home. The contract is an important business tool that is widely used and clearly understood by the people in charge of the nursing home or other long-term care facility.

The contract has several essential parts. The title should simply reflect the purpose of the contract, for example, "Clinical Consultant Agreement." The first paragraph should state the date of the agreement, which can be the date the service described therein begins. The first paragraph also should state the two parties involved in the contract, specifically the name of the long-term care facility, the name of the psychiatric consultant or group, and the addresses of both parties. The second paragraph should state the length of time of the agreement, usually 1 year, and should have some terms regarding the process of termination by either party (e.g., with 30-day written notice).

The third paragraph should outline specific duties and obligations of the consulting psychiatrist and his or her staff. Examples include 24-hours-per-day, 7-days-per-week emergency coverage; the ability of the long-term care facility to reach the consultant by beeper or answering service; the expected schedule of regular rounds by the consultant and his or her staff; and any requirement that the consultant attend quarterly staff meetings, provide a certain number of in-service sessions, or attend clinical case conferences.

Another paragraph should state that the consultant and his or her staff are independent contractors and not employees, servants, or agents of the long-term care facility. A statement should be made that all members of the consultant's staff who perform services are properly licensed, certified, or accredited in the state in which the service is performed. A statement should be made that the agreement will be interpreted and governed in accordance with the laws of the state. And a final statement should be made that the contract exists in good faith between the two parties.

Payment and Termination Provisions

According to Medicare regulations, a service provider is not allowed to receive payment in addition to payment received on assignment from Medicare. Because of this rule, the psychiatrist is not allowed to receive payment for clinical consultation or availability to the long-term care facility. No mention of payment for these services should exist in the contract. There are no Health Care Fi-

nancing Administration (HCFA) regulations prohibiting the consultant psychiatrist and his or her staff from providing administrative service to the long-term care facility for a fee (e.g., serving as medical director or psychiatric director or providing other administrative services). The psychiatrist and his or her staff can charge fees and receive payment for these services. The fees must be at a reasonable, hourly rate similar to that charged by the psychiatrist for administrative services elsewhere. These service records should be well documented.

Additional services can include training long-term care facility staff, making in-service presentations, attending meetings to prepare for state surveys of the long-term care facility, attending meetings to set up psychiatric or activity programs for the residents, and spending time on ethics committees or admission and prescreening committees. A psychiatric team can also provide administrative consultative services (i.e., milieu consultation, consultation with regard to appropriateness of potential new admissions and overall facility management). The psychiatrist and his or her staff can provide these services as a package or in portions. The contract can cover any or all parts of the available services. The time spent on all administrative duties should be separate from time spent on clinical duties in the nursing home.

A contract may need to be terminated for a variety of reasons. A consultant who serves a long-term care facility ideally should avoid needing to terminate a contract because of performance issues. If a nursing care facility is dissatisfied with the consultant's services and the issue is not resolved adequately, the facility has a right to terminate the contract, according to the provisions of the contract (e.g., with 30-day written notice). The same is true for a consultant who chooses to terminate the contract. The termination aspect of the contract is simple because the only successful relationship between a consultant and a long-term care facility is one in which there is a mutual wish and desire for the services to be rendered to the facility. If this mutuality breaks down, the consultant cannot serve the long-term care facility well, and the contract provisions should allow for a quick termination of the contract.

Psychiatric services can be provided to the nursing home under an exclusive contract, which means that no other psychiatrist, by contract, can render services in the nursing home. Contracting may be done on a nonexclusive basis, which would allow other like providers to provide parallel psychiatric services, at the request of family, attending physicians, or facility.

The HCFA has addressed mental health services provided in long-term care facilities. Federal law states that in order for a skilled nursing facility to participate in Medicare Part A, it must provide services "necessary to attain or maintain the highest practicable, physical, mental and psychosocial well-being of each resident" (Social Security Act, Section 1819(b)(4)(A)). This means that in order to receive reimbursement from Medicare for services (e.g., daily rate of nursing home, rehabilitation, pharmacy), the nursing home is required to provide treatment for mental health problems. The psychiatrist is in a unique position to contract with the nursing home to provide these services. The psychiatrist is not allowed to provide money or gifts to the nursing home in exchange for these referrals. In addition, he or she is not allowed to receive payment from the nursing home for the treatment of these patients, as these services should be billed to Medicare Part B.

As mentioned in Chapter 6, the Balanced Budget Act of 1997 includes a consolidated billing requirement. Although the regulations will not be implemented fully until July 2000, one provision of the new regulations is already in effect. Nursing homes are now required to provide licensed clinical social worker (LCSW) services to Medicare Part A skilled nursing home patients under the new prospective payment system. Because the nursing homes are required by law to provide mental health services, those nursing homes that do not directly employ social workers may want to contract with the psychiatrist for these services.

In summary, the written contract between the psychiatrist and nursing home may be used to cement a long-lasting, mutually beneficial relationship. This chapter has outlined various types of contracts and updated the reader on HCFA regulations regarding mental health services to nursing homes.

References

Social Security Act, Section 1819(b)(4)(A)

Tariot PN, Podgorski CA, Blazina L, et al: Mental disorders in the nursing home: another perspective. Am J Psychiatry 150:1063–1069, 1993

Section 4

Legal and Ethical Issues

Chapter 8

Legal and Ethical Issues

In this chapter we offer a topical and clinically focused discussion of the legal and ethical issues that arise in providing psychiatric treatment to nursing home patients. We do not offer a comprehensive theory of clinical ethics or a complete review of the subject. Other relevant topics include restraint use, sexuality and privacy issues, and criteria for involuntary nursing home commitment (which vary on the state level). Comprehensive information on these important topics may be found elsewhere (Barnett 1978; Burton et al. 1990; Fletcher 1996; Lyder 1994; Margolis et al. 1986; Marks 1992; McCartney et al. 1994; Miles and Irvine 1992; Richardson and Lazur 1995; Tinetti et al. 1992).

Psychiatrists may function in two major kinds of consulting roles in the nursing home setting. Traditionally they respond to cases referred from primary care physicians. Alternatively they may be retained as ongoing consultants to residents and staff of a long-term care facility.

The psychiatrist who is a consultant in a long-term care setting, where 80%–90% of residents may have a secondary psychiatric diagnosis, has complex ethical duties related to the general nature of the nursing home environment (Rovner et al. 1990; Tariot et al. 1993). First, the consultant faces the dehumanization implicit in the diagnostic or labeling use of terms such as "wanderer," "uncooperative," or "assaultive." Such behavioral descriptors can sometimes divert attention away from underlying etiologies or, worse, lead to stigmatization as exemplified by the abusive or even punitive use of restraints (Berland et al. 1990; Schnelle et al. 1992). Second,

some ethics issues are taken for granted by nursing home staff but are of great importance to nursing home residents. These issues include regulations about bedtimes, rising times, bath times, and meal times; roommate choice; sexual life; private telephone access; passes to leave the facility; and rules regarding liquor (Ambrogi 1989; Hofland 1988; Kane and Caplan 1990). The scale of personal control in a total-care institution such as a nursing home is often needlessly dehumanizing. This is an important theme for a psychiatric consultant to address. To engage these issues, the psychiatrist will have to participate in education at all levels of the facility's staff and administration, including the medical director and the resident's primary care physicians. When available, consultation with an in-house ethics committee or a geriatric psychiatrist concerning specific legal and ethical issues is always indicated.

Nursing Home Placement

Nursing home placement entails a radical change in a patient's definition of self and in others' perceptions of the patient. Fear of nursing home placement is a common precipitant of suicide (Loebel et al. 1991). Nursing home placement can disrupt the conduct of marital and social relationships and impoverish the patient, a noninstitutionalized spouse, or other family members. These possible consequences of nursing home placements justify a high standard of patient advocacy on the part of psychiatrists involved in these decisions. First, diligent efforts must be made to keep the patient at home by optimizing his or her biopsychosocial functioning through both health and social services. Second, supportive counseling should be available for persons who are at risk for nursing home placement. Finally, placement decisions should be based on a demonstrated, rather than predicted, failure to be able to care for one's self. Proper legal authority should be required in order to institutionalize a person who is opposed to needed nursing home placement.

Competence and Decision-Making Ability

Psychiatrists are often asked to assess a patient's decision-making capacity; to assess the authenticity of a patient's particular decision; or to recommend a decision-making process for a person who is unable to make decisions. This may occur when a patient refuses a recommended medical treatment (e.g., antidepressants and other medications, life-sustaining care); when a caregiver can no longer manage a patient (e.g., when a frail person who is unable to live in the community refuses home care or nursing home placement); or when a family caregiver disagrees with a patient's decision (e.g., when a dementia patient decides to continue driving). When a request for psychiatric consultation regarding treatment refusal raises a question of the patient's decision-making capacity, the patient may have organic mental disease or alcoholism or other problems that can adversely affect the patient's ability to live independently (Golinger and Federoff 1989; Mahler et al. 1990; Mebane and Rauch 1990). By contrast, when a patient's decision-making ability is not challenged in a psychiatric consultation for treatment refusal, the dispute about the treatment in question can often be resolved successfully by brief counseling that focuses on the situational reasons for the refusal (Howanitz and Freedman 1992).

Competence, decision-making ability, and informed consent are different concepts. Competence, or incompetence, is a legal status. Incompe-

tence is a court finding that places a person under the legal control of a court-appointed guardian. By contrast, decision-making ability is a clinical finding. Although these terms are often used interchangeably, the difference between them emphasizes the limited authority of a clinician over patients who have not been declared incompetent, and the definitive authority of a designated guardian for a person who has been found incompetent. Moreover, both of these terms differ from a forensic finding of responsibility for a crime.

For decision-making ability to be present, a patient must be able to 1) receive and communicate information, even after attempts to reverse or overcome sensory or speech disorders have failed; 2) appreciate the personal implications, both short and long term, of risks and benefits; and 3) provide a cogent explanation of how he or she weighs the risks and benefits or relates them to personal goals. The clinical conclusion that a patient lacks decision-making ability may lead to the decision to seek a legal finding that a patient is incompetent and in need of a legal guardian. The guardian's responsibility is to make appropriate decisions about health care issues that are in the best interests of the patient. These could include using emergency medical holds or treatment powers; using a proxy decision maker named in an advance directive; or perhaps deciding to use certain human services, such as nursing home placement or a home-health professional, to dispense medications.

Decision making should be assessed as a process, rather than simply in relation to the perceived strangeness of a patient's particular decision. Thus a patient's decision making should not be deemed impaired simply because it is unusual, or even unreasonable, or because the decision is supported by unconventional premises. However, patients should be able to give an account of their decision making, describing the major grounds for a decision and relating the decision to those grounds. Major decisions also should not change arbitrarily, although they may evolve with further discussion or experience or in relation to the manner in which the issue or information is framed.

Decision-making incapacity may be limited in time and scope. It may be transient and reversible when caused by medical conditions (e.g., delirium), social situations (e.g., learned dependence), or risk-averse life orientations or when a person is temporarily overwhelmed by an unfamiliar or catastrophic situation. Decision-making incapacity may also be limited to a small set of decisions. For example, a patient may be unable to evaluate a particular treatment, while being fully capable of deciding that a daughter, rather than a spouse, should be the proxy decision maker. Similarly, a patient may need a financial conservator even though otherwise capable of making his or her own medical decisions and living independently.

The doctrine of informed consent holds that a patient, or proxy with decision-making capacity, must be given sufficient information and the freedom to make an authentic treatment decision. Patients should be given information that will be germane to how they make decisions. This includes information on why a therapy is proposed, the likelihood of benefit, the incidence and range of undesirable side effects, and alternatives to the recommended course. Germane information needs to be defined in relation to the patient's values. For example, when obtaining consent to remove a colonic polyp from a patient who is a Jehovah's Witness with a strong, religiously grounded objection to receiving blood, the physician should discuss with the patient the rare possibility of a blood transfusion.

Forgoing Life-Sustaining Treatment

Psychiatrists become involved in decisions to withdraw or withhold life-sustaining treatment when they are asked to 1) evaluate a patient's decision-making capacity; 2) assess whether depressive or other psychiatric symptoms are influencing the patient's decision making; and 3) counsel patients and families about decisions to forgo treatment. The withdrawal or withholding of life-sustaining treatment precedes about 1.5 million deaths in the United States each year (about

75% of hospital inpatient deaths and a higher percentage of nursing home deaths). Half of these patients do not make the decision to withdraw or withhold treatment, often because clinicians have deferred discussing this issue, thus passing decisions on to family members.

A legal and clinical standard of care exists for these decisions (Council on Ethics and Judicial Affairs 1992; Meisel 1991). This standard includes the following principles:

- All life-sustaining treatments are elective.
- Medically provided food and fluid are life-sustaining treatments.
- Consent must be obtained, for any life-sustaining treatment, from the patient or a person who can speak for the patient's interests.
- The right to consent to or refuse treatment is not conditional on having a terminal or irreversible illness.

States vary as to the degree of proof that they require as evidence of an incompetent person's preference to forgo treatment. States also vary in procedures pertaining to the selection and empowerment of proxy decision makers and with regard to decisions for persons under state guardianship or in state-owned health-care facilities. Court involvement is rare—about 100 Appeals Court decisions have been made since 1976. Patients usually perceive discussions with physicians about the limited use of life-sustaining treatments as positive experiences; these discussions address patients' fears, give them a sense of being cared for, and decrease depressive symptoms (Finucane et al. 1988; Kellogg et al. 1992; Lo et al. 1986; Stolman et al. 1990). A small number of patients find this counseling to be upsetting or saddening, or develop a sense of resignation or health-related fear. Successful counseling focuses on enhancement of the patient's sense of control and on the goal of continuing the treatment relationship. Counseling must avoid the implicit suggestion that the patient is being abandoned, which can arise if the discussion is focused on the limitation of treatment.

Psychiatrists participating in these decisions should address both the affective and cognitive components of decision making. They should consider the possibility of depression, under-treated (often chronic) pain, adjustment disorders to catastrophic illness, or other factors that might affect a patient's request to forgo life-sustaining treatment. Depressive symptoms alone, as opposed to a diagnosis of a clinical depressive disorder, do not disqualify or appear to affect these decisions (Cohen-Mansfield et al. 1991; Shmerling et al. 1988). For example, older patients' preferences for cardiopulmonary resuscitation (CPR) are influenced by their overly optimistic estimate of the efficacy of resuscitation. About one in seven persons who receives CPR while in the hospital survives to discharge; this number decreases substantially when cardiac arrest occurs in patients who are chronically ill or have multiorgan system disease. Survival after nursing home resuscitation is very rare. These realistic outcomes should be discussed empathetically with patients in the course of counseling them about treatment plans.

Physicians should encourage patients to make advance directives to clarify future decisions about life-sustaining treatment, in the event that the patient loses decision-making capacity. A *living will* specifies an individual's values and preferences for medical care. One form of living will creates a values history, in which personal questions in everyday language define the patient's values; these values should guide the patient's medical care (Lambert et al. 1990). Other living wills require the individual to choose treatments for hypothetical terminal illness, coma, or dementia (Emaneul and Emaneul 1992). This format offers clinicians more specific guidance about the patient's wishes but uses more technical medical language.

A *durable power of attorney* for health care enables an individual to appoint someone to make treatment choices in the event of his or her loss of decision-making ability. In effect, this enables a person to appoint his or her own guardian. A durable power of attorney is particularly useful when a person wants an unrelated friend or a distant relative to supersede the immediate family.

Durable power of attorney has an advantage over a living will in that it empowers a person who can interpret the patient's past statements and values (Annas 1991). Most people want living wills interpreted flexibly (Sehgal et al. 1992). Studies show that surrogate decision makers, including physicians, have a very limited ability to estimate exactly a person's treatment preferences (Seckler et al. 1991).

Proxy decision makers should be chosen on the basis of their intimate familiarity with the patient's values rather than simply on the basis of the closeness of their kinship, as is done when identifying individuals to consent to autopsies or organ donation. Proxy decision makers should be encouraged to discuss the patient's preferences for care rather than their own.

Comfort Care for Patients With End-Stage Dementia

Comfort care for patients with profound dementia is similar to other forms of hospice care. It rests on the foundation of a thorough medical evaluation and conscientious decision making about treatment goals (Miles and Moss 1988). Comfort care may be based on an advance directive or on the conclusion that the patient is not experiencing the benefit of life-sustaining therapy that is being provided. It may follow a recognition that a patient is anorexic and that life-sustaining food or fluids could be provided only by the unacceptable use of permanent enteral nutrition. It is usually possible to conduct family meetings in these situations to arrive at a reasonable consensus between health-care providers and family members (Volicer et al. 1986). Like discussions with patients, such family counseling should be based on how the patient will be cared for and on the patient's interests. Such positive foundations give an essential context to family members, who otherwise may feel that they are being asked to abandon a loved one.

A comfort-care-only treatment plan entails a comprehensive review of medications and therapies. Routine laboratory tests or medications that prolong life but do not comfort (e.g., antiarrhythmics, lipid-lowering agents) are not indicated. Life-sustaining medications may be appropriate if they minimize suffering (e.g., diuretics for congestive heart failure). Calorie counts are misleading in patients who are expected to die and who have refused a feeding tube; the chart should note that patients have been offered food or fluids to satisfy their hunger or thirst. Other measures, such as physical therapies, skin care, and new hearing aid batteries, should be provided as needed to optimize quality of life and always to prevent suffering. Hospitalization is ordinarily not indicated except for palliative treatment that is beyond the capability of the long-term facility. If a patient is transferred to a hospital, especially via an ambulance, the physician should ensure that the comfort-care-only treatment plan is transmitted to the ambulance attendants, emergency department staff, and inpatient providers (Sachs et al. 1991).

Truth Telling and the Diagnosis of Alzheimer's Disease

The diagnosis of Alzheimer's disease has profound implications for both patients and their caregivers. Besides being a grave condition in itself, the diagnosis can affect how a person is perceived by others. It can affect the price of, or even the patient's ability to purchase, health and long-term care insurance. It can also affect admission to some retirement facilities, authority over personal affairs, and the standing of wills and contracts. Emerging genetic testing may eventually enable clinicians to predict whether a patient has a high likelihood of acquiring Alzheimer's disease, assuming that death from other causes does not occur in the time between the test and old age.

It is currently obligatory to tell patients of diagnoses. One study has shown that more than 90% of adults would want to be told of the diagnosis of Alzheimer's disease in order to be able to make plans for their own care, to settle family and business matters, and to obtain a second opinion (Erde

et al. 1988). People with early Alzheimer's disease can be harmed by not being told. They may be deprived of the opportunity to make a will, to appoint a proxy decision maker, or to leave instructions for their family. The uncertain nature of most early Alzheimer's disease diagnoses is part of this important information. In order to respect patients and enhance their choices, they should be told of this diagnosis as they would be told of any other.

The Role of Caregivers

Psychiatrists, especially those who work in nursing home settings, will meet former and current caregivers for many frail, disabled, or cognitively impaired older patients. These caregivers play complex roles in the lives of older persons. They often have a unique, intimate, and long-standing relationship with the patient, attending and sometimes speaking for the patient during encounters with medical and nursing staff, social workers, physical therapists, and even other visiting family members.

The most powerful role of former caregivers in a nursing-home setting is as proxy decision makers when a patient has impaired decision-making ability. They often are asked to ratify (and thus are also empowered to veto) decisions for incompetent patients. Numerous studies show that a proxy decision maker's decisions correlate imperfectly with the patient's own views and may overestimate, for example, the degree of aggressive treatment an elderly patient who has dementia or is unconscious would want (Danis et al. 1991; Tomlinson et al. 1990; Zweibel and Cassel 1989). There is no consensus on how best to clinically manage such situations, although the ethical consensus is that the decision should center on the patient's preferences and values. A psychiatrist in this situation may help a caregiver become more aware of how the caregiver's own emotions may be affecting the decisions and also may help the caregiver sort out the patient's interests from the caregiver's own needs and fears.

References

Ambrogi DM: Legal issues in nursing home admissions. Law, Medicine and Health Care 18:254–262, 1989

Annas GJ: The health care proxy and the living will. N Engl J Med 324:1210–1213, 1991

Barnett CF: Treatment rights of mentally ill nursing home residents. University of Pennsylvania Law Review 126:578–629, 1978

Berland B, Wachtel TJ, Kiel DP, et al: Patient characteristics associated with the use of mechanical restraints. J Gen Intern Med 5:480–484, 1990

Burton LC, German PS, Rovner BW, et al: Mental illness and the use of restraints in nursing homes. J Gen Intern Med 5:480–485, 1990

Cohen-Mansfield J, Rabinovich BA, Lipson S, et al: The decision to execute a durable power of attorney for health care and preferences regarding the use of life-sustaining treatments in nursing home residents. Arch Intern Med 151:289–294, 1991

Council on Ethics and Judicial Affairs: Decisions near the end of life. JAMA 267:2229–2233, 1992

Danis M, Southerland LI, Garrett JM, et al: A prospective study of advance directives for life-sustaining care. N Engl J Med 234:882–888, 1991

Emaneul LL, Emaneul EJ: The medical directive: a new comprehensive advance care document. JAMA 267:2229–2233, 1992

Erde E, Nodal E, Scholl T: On truth-telling and the diagnosis of Alzheimer's disease. J Fam Pract 26:401–403, 1988

Finucane TE, Shumway JM, Powers RL, et al: Planning with elderly outpatients for contingencies of severe illness: a survey and clinical trial. J Gen Intern Med 2:322–325, 1988

Fletcher K: Use of restraints in the elderly. American Association of Critical-Care Nurses Clinical Issues 7(4):611–635, 1996

Golinger RC, Federoff JP: Characteristics of patients referred to psychiatrists for competency evaluations. Psychosomatics 30:296–299, 1989

Hofland BF (ed): Autonomy and long-term care. Gerontologist 28 (suppl):2–96, 1988

Howanitz EM, Freedman JB: Reasons for refusal of medical treatment by patients seen by a consultation-liaison service. Hosp Community Psychiatry 43:278–279, 1992

Kane RA, Caplan AL (eds): Everyday Ethics: Resolving Dilemmas in Nursing Home Life. New York, Springer, 1990

Kellogg FR, Crain M, Corwin J, et al: Life-sustaining interventions in frail elderly persons: talking about choices. Arch Intern Med 152:2317–2320, 1992

Lambert JP, Gibson JM, Nathanson P: Values history: an innovation in surrogate medical decision making. Law, Medicine and Health Care 18:202–212, 1990

Lo B, McLeod GA, Saika G: Patient attitudes to discussion of life-sustaining treatments. Arch Gen Intern Med 146:1613–1615, 1986

Loebel JP, Loebel J, Dager SR, et al: Anticipation of nursing home placement may be a precipitant of suicide among the elderly. J Am Geriatr Soc 39:407–408, 1991

Lyder CH: The role of the nurse practitioner in promoting sexuality in the institutionalized elderly. Journal of the American Academy of Nurse Practitioners 6:61–63, 1994

Mahler JC, Perry S, Miller F: Psychiatric evaluation of competency in physically ill patients who refuse treatment. Hosp Community Psychiatry 41:1140–1141, 1990

Margolis EJ, Barry PP, Markson LJ, et al: Institutionalizing the elderly involuntarily: how far can you go? Geriatrics 41:89–92, 94–95, 1986

Marks W: Physical restraints in the practice of medicine: current concepts. Arch Intern Med 152:2203–2206, 1992

McCartney JR, Izeman H, Rogers D, et al: Sexuality and the institutionalized elderly. J Am Geriatr Soc 35:61–63, 1994

Mebane AH, Rauch HB: When do physicians request competency evaluations? Psychosomatics 31:40–46, 1990

Meisel A: Legal myths about terminating life support. Arch Gen Intern Med 151:1497–1502, 1991

Miles SH, Irvine P: Deaths caused by physical restraints. Gerontologist 32:762–766, 1992

Miles SH, Moss R: Evaluating life-sustaining treatments for demented patients. Clin Geriatr Med 4:917–924, 1988

Richardson JP, Lazur A: Sexuality in the nursing home patient. Am Fam Physician 51:121–124, 1995

Rovner B, German P, Broadhead J, et al: Prevalence and management of dementia and other psychiatric disorders in nursing homes. Int Psychogeriatr 2:13, 1990

Sachs GA, Miles SH, Levin R: Limiting resuscitation: emerging policy in the emergency medical system. Ann Intern Med 114:151–154, 1991

Schnelle JF, Simmons SF, Ory MG: Risk factor that predict staff failure to release nursing home residents from restraints. Gerontologist 32:767–770, 1992

Seckler AB, Meier DE, Mulvihill M, et al: Substituted judgment: how accurate are proxy predictions? Ann Intern Med 115:92–98,1991

Sehgal A, Galbraith A, Chesney M, et al: How strictly do dialysis patients want their advance directives followed? JAMA 267:59–63, 1992

Shmerling RH, Bedell S, Lilienfield A, et al: Discussing cardiopulmonary resuscitation: a study of elderly outpatients. J Gen Intern Med 3:317–321, 1988

Stolman CJ, Gregory JJ, Dunn D, et al: Evaluation of patient, physician, nurse and family attitudes toward do-not-resuscitate orders. Arch Intern Med 150:653–658, 1990

Tariot PN, Podgorski CA, Blazina L, et al: Mental disorders in the nursing home: another perspective. Am J Psychiatry 150:1063–1069, 1993

Tinetti ME, Liu WL, Ginter SF: Mechanical restraint use and fall-related injuries among residents of skilled nursing facilities. Ann Intern Med 116:369–374, 1992

Tomlinson T, Howe K, Notman M, et al: An empirical study of proxy consent for elderly persons. Gerontologist 30:54–64, 1990

Volicer L, Rheaume Y, Brown J, et al: Hospice approach to the treatment of patients with advanced dementia of the Alzheimer type. JAMA 256:2210–2213, 1986

Zweibel NR, Cassel CK: Treatment choices at the end of life: a comparison of decisions by older patients and their physicians, selected proxies. Gerontologist 29:615–621, 1989

Section 5

Perspectives for the Future

Chapter 9

Perspectives for the Future

Ideally the psychiatrist can develop a decision tree or algorithm for identifying, assessing, consulting on, and providing treatment to patients in nursing homes. Also, resources must be better utilized by psychiatrists. For example, providers of outpatient mental health services must be paid more equitably in order to effect long-term improvement in the system.

The best model for the improved diagnosis and treatment of mental illness among nursing home patients is one in which all mental health providers work together with an emphasis on a full continuum-of-care model that utilizes both medical and psychosocial theory and practice.

Managed care cost-containment solutions and federal regulations such as Omnibus Reconciliation Act of 1987 (OBRA-87) have had the perhaps unintended effect of dictating physician care. For various reasons most psychiatrists and other physicians are allowing policies, legislation, and protocols to be decided largely by others.

The American Psychiatric Association, the American Association for Geriatric Psychiatry, and the Geriatric Psychiatry Alliance are positioned to proceed beyond the current series of seminars to educate one another and our colleagues. These organizations represent the only significant voices we have in addressing the future need for psychiatric involvement in the nursing home and in other health-care arenas. We need to develop a vision for where we wish to be 10, 20, and 30 years from now. We need to learn that current social evolutionary processes have dictated our present status. We do not have to accept that this is inevitable. We have the knowledge base via neuropsychiatry and biomedical re-search to establish the link between physical and mental health. We have the expertise to help people cope better to prevent disease. We should be using our financial and knowledge base resources to build future systems based on a psycho-biosocial treatment and educational approach.

Until the medical and social models are better integrated, psychiatric care in nursing homes will be guided largely by current sociopolitical and financial forces created to reduce spending in all health care (i.e., managed care, block grants, and funding cuts). Improvement in psychiatric care in nursing homes can be achieved in the next 10–15 years if

- The role of the psychiatrist is developed as the "captain" of the nursing home treatment team. The solution for the immediate future may best be represented by the consultation-liaison model. Psychiatrists need to own their responsibility for a commitment to a well-functioning multidisciplinary team, which recent studies show can provide the best, most efficient, and least expensive high-quality service to long-term care patients.

- Critical pathways (algorithms) are developed to better define psychiatric assessment and treatment services.

- All psychiatrists own their responsibility for good geriatric training and do not assume that such training should be limited to specialists in geriatric psychiatry.

- Psychiatrists commit energy to influence the political process by working through psychiatric organizations.

Appendixes

Appendix A

Staffing in Long-Term Care

Staffing in long-term care facilities involves a variety of professionals and nonprofessionals. This appendix contains a list of the main staff members with descriptions of their roles and responsibilities.

Activity director. The activity director is responsible for developing and implementing appropriate activities that will enhance the residents' well-being. Activity programs are mandated by law and are intertwined with social services. These programs are designed to appropriately meet the needs and interests of the residents, encourage their self-care and resumption of normal activities, and achieve an optimal level of psychological functioning.

Administrator. The administrator is in charge of the facility's day-to-day operations. He or she is responsible for the level of health care the patients receive, the safety of the patients, and the protection of their personal rights and property. The administrator also makes facility policy, supervises personnel, and handles fiscal matters.

Admissions director. The admissions director is responsible for keeping up the census in a facility. He or she works with discharge planners at hospitals, meets with prospective new residents and families, and makes presentations in the community about the facility's services.

Audiologist/speech therapist. The audiologist/ speech therapist works most often with residents who have experienced a hearing loss, stroke, or other ailment affecting their hearing and speech. These services are utilized as needed to help patients improve and maintain their functioning.

Certified nurse's assistant. A certified nurse's assistant, or nurse's aide, provides most of the care to nursing home residents. He or she is responsible for taking care of the residents' day-to-day basic needs. Aides receive some minimum training, but their work is best learned through on-the-job training. These workers are underpaid, overworked, and often not appreciated. Regular continuing education must be provided because of high turnover.

Charge nurse. To qualify as a charge nurse, one must be a registered nurse or a qualified licensed practical or vocational nurse. The charge nurse supervises all nursing activities on his or her shift. Charge nurses supervise the other nurses and aides, provide hands-on physical care of residents, act as a liaison with other professionals, and talk with family members. At least one registered nurse must be employed during every day shift. Licensed nursing services must be provided around the clock.

Dietitian. The dietitian ensures that the food meets the residents' daily nutritional and special dietary needs. The meals are also supposed to be attractive and palatable. Patients who require assistance in eating must receive this service.

Director of nurses. The director of nurses is a qualified nurse, employed full time, who has administrative authority, responsibility, and accountability for the functions, activities, and training of the nursing services staff. The director is the manager of patient care.

Family council. The family council comprises a group of family members of residents. They usually meet on a monthly basis to provide support for one another and discuss concerns about the residents and the facility.

Housekeeping. The housekeeping staff keeps the physical plant clean and safe. (They can be among the best referral sources.)

Medical director. The medical director is employed by the facility on either a part-time or full-time basis as needed. He or she has overall responsibility for the patients' medical care. The director also reviews all admissions, makes recommendations on patient care policy, and monitors the quality of care.

Occupational therapist. The occupational therapist works with residents to help them regain or maintain their activities of daily living.

Pharmacy consultant. The pharmacy consultant develops, coordinates, and supervises all pharmaceutical services. He or she reviews drug regimens for each resident monthly and reports to the medical director and administrator any discrepancies or irregularities. The pharmacy consultant develops procedures for control and accountability of all drugs and biological agents throughout the facility. The overall pharmaceutical service develops written policies and procedures for safe and effective drug therapy.

Physical therapist. An important member of the rehabilitation team, the physical therapist is re-

sponsible for patient rehabilitation and restoration of functioning. Residents recovering from a stroke or serious injury are prime candidates. Physical therapy services are used widely in long-term care facilities. Therapists provide valuable and needed assistance in maintaining residents' level of functioning and in preventing further deterioration.

Primary care physician. Each resident is assigned a primary care physician. By law, a resident must be examined within 48 hours of admission, every 30 days for the first 90 days in residence, and at least once every 90 days thereafter.

Program/staff developer. The program/staff developer facilitates education programs for the nursing staff. He or she provides training for the certified nurse's assistants/nurse's aides and often brings in outside professionals to help with these programs. The developer also provides continuing education to the staff.

Resident council. Similar to a family council, the resident council is made up of a group of residents who meet monthly to discuss problems and concerns. These groups are usually led by the activity or social services director. They usually have little effect on policy.

Social services designee. Any facility that has more than 120 beds must have a full-time social services designee. The designee often works with residents and their families to ensure that resident rights are protected. He or she works with hospital discharge planners upon the resident's admission to the facility and develops discharge plans for the resident when he or she is discharged. The social services designee also provides psychosocial care.

Appendix B

Sample Preadmission Note to a Nursing Home

Dear Colleagues:

My patient, _____, will soon be admitted to your facility. To help you plan his/her care, I have attached an admission Minimum Data Set form, partially filled out based on my most recent assessment and on input from the family and the other clinicians involved with the case. The assessment was completed on

_____.

   After _____ is admitted, I would appreciate your faxing me a copy of your admission treatment plan. If you wish to discuss any aspect of his/her case with me in connection with planning the treatment, the best way to reach me is _____.

   A brief summary of my psychiatric assessment and treatment recommendations is found on the following page.

Psychiatric diagnosis:

Medical/neurological conditions or current medications affecting psychiatric status:

Recommended psychotropic medication:

Recommended nonpharmacologic treatment or management:

Potential behavioral emergencies and recommended response:

Suggested monitoring method and schedule:

Expected date of first psychiatric visit to the patient after admission to your facility:

Appendix C

Sample Form for Transfer From a Nursing Home to a Hospital or Clinic

Dear Colleagues:

Our patient, _____, will soon be admitted to your facility. To help you plan his/her care, we have attached an admission Minimum Data Set (MDS) form, plus an update of the MDS based on his/her most recent assessment, completed on _____.

We encourage you to use the MDS as a reference regarding the patient's baseline functional and cognitive status and regarding his/her legal status advance directives for medical treatment. If any part of the MDS is unclear to you, please contact _____ at our facility (telephone: _____) and your questions will be answered.

An outline of essential points is found on the following page.

The patient's legal status:

Advance directives limiting medical treatment:

Baseline of physical and cognitive function when the patient was last medically stable:

Psychiatric and behavioral issues, with recommended management:

Psychotropic medications:

Diagnostic questions and issues about which we would like your opinion:

Appendix D

MINIMUM DATA SET (MDS) — *VERSION 2.0*
FOR NURSING HOME RESIDENT ASSESSMENT AND CARE SCREENING
BASIC ASSESSMENT TRACKING FORM

SECTION AA. IDENTIFICATION INFORMATION		GENERAL INSTRUCTIONS

GENERAL INSTRUCTIONS

Complete this information for submission with all full and quarterly assessments (Admission, Annual, Significant Change, State or Medicare required assessments, or Quarterly Reviews, etc.).

1. RESIDENT NAME ⊛
a. (First)　　b. (Middle Initial)　　c. (Last)　　d. (Jr./Sr.)

2. GENDER ⊛
1. Male　　2. Female

3. BIRTHDATE ⊛
Month — Day — Year

4. RACE/ETHNICITY ⊛
1. American Indian/Alaskan Native
2. Asian/Pacific Islander
3. Black, not of Hispanic origin
4. Hispanic
5. White, not of Hispanic origin

5. SOCIAL SECURITY ⊛ AND ⊛ MEDICARE NUMBERS [C in 1st box if non Med. no.]
a. Social Security Number

b. Medicare number (or comparable railroad insurance number)

6. FACILITY PROVIDER NO. ⊛
a. State No.

b. Federal No.

7. MEDICAID NO. ["+" if pending, "N" if not a Medicaid ⊛ recipient]

8. REASONS FOR ASSESSMENT
[Note—Other codes do not apply to this form]
a. Primary reason for assessment
  1. Admission assessment (required by day 14)
  2. Annual assessment
  3. Significant change in status assessment
  4. Significant correction of prior assessment
  5. Quarterly review assessment
  0. *NONE OF ABOVE*
b. *Special codes for use with supplemental assessment types in Case Mix demonstration states or other states where required*
  1. 5 day assessment
  2. 30 day assessment
  3. 60 day assessment
  4. Quarterly assessment using full MDS form
  5. Readmission/return assessment
  6. Other state required assessment

9. SIGNATURES OF PERSONS COMPLETING THESE ITEMS:

a. Signatures　　Title　　Date

b.　　Date

⊛ = Key items for computerized resident tracking

▨ = When box blank, must enter number or letter

[a.] = When letter in box, check if condition applies

Code "NA" if information unavailable or unknown.

TRIGGER LEGEND

1 - Delirium	**10A** - Activities (Revise)
2 - Cognitive Loss/Dementia	**10B** - Activities (Review)
3 - Visual Function	**11** - Falls
4 - Communication	**12** - Nutritional Status
5A - ADL-Rehabilitation	**13** - Feeding Tubes
5B - ADL-Maintenance	**14** - Dehydration/Fluid Maintenance
6 - Urinary Incontinence and Indwelling Catheter	**15** - Dental Care
7 - Psychosocial Well-Being	**16** - Pressure Ulcers
8 - Mood State	**17** - Psychotropic Drug Use
9 - Behavioral Symptoms	**17*** - For this to trigger, O4a, b, or c must = 1-7
	18 - Physical Restraints

Form 1728HF　© 1995 Briggs Corporation, Des Moines, IA 50306 (800) 247-2343 PRINTED IN U.S.A.
R196　　Copyright limited to addition of trigger system.

1 of 8

MDS 2.0　10/18/94N

Resident _____ Numeric Identifier _____

MINIMUM DATA SET (MDS) — *VERSION 2.0*
FOR NURSING HOME RESIDENT ASSESSMENT AND CARE SCREENING
BACKGROUND (FACE SHEET) INFORMATION AT ADMISSION

SECTION AB. DEMOGRAPHIC INFORMATION

1.	DATE OF ENTRY	Date the stay began. Note — Does not include readmission if record was closed at time of temporary discharge to hospital, etc. In such cases, use prior admission date.

☐☐ — ☐☐ — ☐☐☐☐
Month   Day   Year

2.	ADMITTED FROM (AT ENTRY)	1. Private home/apt. with no home health services 2. Private home/apt. with home health services 3. Board and care/assisted living/group home 4. Nursing home 5. Acute care hospital 6. Psychiatric hospital, MR/DD facility 7. Rehabilitation hospital 8. Other
3.	LIVED ALONE (PRIOR TO ENTRY)	0. No 1. Yes 2. In other facility
4.	ZIP CODE OF PRIOR PRIMARY RESIDENCE	☐☐☐☐☐

5. RESIDENTIAL HISTORY 5 YEARS PRIOR TO ENTRY — *(Check all settings resident lived in during 5 years prior to date of entry given in item AB1 above.)*

Prior stay at this nursing home	a.
Stay in other nursing home	b.
Other residential facility — board and care home, assisted living, group home	c.
MH/psychiatric setting	d.
MR/DD setting	e.
NONE OF ABOVE	f.

6.	LIFETIME OCCUPA-TION(S) (Put "/" between two occupations)	☐☐☐☐☐☐☐☐☐☐☐☐☐☐☐
7.	EDUCATION (Highest level completed)	1. No schooling 5. Technical or trade school 2. 8th grade/less 6. Some college 3. 9-11 grades 7. Bachelor's degree 4. High school 8. Graduate degree
8.	LANGUAGE	(Code for correct response) a. Primary Language 0. English 1. Spanish 2. French 3. Other
		b. If other, specify ☐☐☐☐☐☐☐☐
9.	MENTAL HEALTH HISTORY	Does resident's RECORD indicate any history of mental retardation, mental illness, or developmental disability problem? 0. No 1. Yes

10. CONDITIONS RELATED TO MR/DD STATUS — *(Check all conditions that are related to MR/DD status that were manifested before age 22, and are likely to continue indefinitely)*

Not applicable — no MR/DD (Skip to AB11)	a.
MR/DD with organic condition	
Down's syndrome	b.
Autism	c.
Epilepsy	d.
Other organic condition related to MR/DD	e.
MR/DD with no organic condition	f.

11.	DATE BACK-GROUND INFORMA-TION COMPLETED	☐☐ — ☐☐ — ☐☐☐☐ Month Day Year

▨ = When box blank, must enter number or letter

☐a. = When letter in box, check if condition applies

Code "NA" if information unavailable or unknown.

SECTION AC. CUSTOMARY ROUTINE

1. CUSTOMARY ROUTINE *(In year prior to DATE OF ENTRY to this nursing home, or year last in community if now being admitted from another nursing home)* — *(Check all that apply. If all information UNKNOWN, check last box only.)*

CYCLE OF DAILY EVENTS	
Stays up late at night (e.g., after 9 pm)	a.
Naps regularly during day (at least 1 hour)	b.
Goes out 1+ days a week	c.
Stays busy with hobbies, reading, or fixed daily routine	d.
Spends most of time alone or watching TV	e.
Moves independently indoors (with appliances, if used)	f.
Use of tobacco products at least daily	g.
NONE OF ABOVE	h.
EATING PATTERNS	
Distinct food preferences	i.
Eats between meals all or most days	j.
Use of alcoholic beverage(s) at least weekly	k.
NONE OF ABOVE	l.
ADL PATTERNS	
In bedclothes much of day	m.
Wakens to toilet all or most nights	n.
Has irregular bowel movement pattern	o.
Showers for bathing	p.
Bathing in PM	q.
NONE OF ABOVE	r.
INVOLVEMENT PATTERNS	
Daily contact with relatives/close friends	s.
Usually attends church, temple, synagogue (etc.)	t.
Finds strength in faith	u.
Daily animal companion/presence	v.
Involved in group activities	w.
NONE OF ABOVE	x.
UNKNOWN — Resident/family unable to provide information	y.

☐ **END**

SECTION AD. FACE SHEET SIGNATURES

SIGNATURES OF PERSONS COMPLETING FACE SHEET:

a. Signature of RN Assessment Coordinator			Date
b. Signatures	Title	Sections	Date
c.			Date
d.			Date
e.			Date
f.			Date
g.			Date

NOTE: Normally, the MDS Face Sheet is completed once, when an individual first enters the facility. However, the face sheet is also required if the person is reentering this facility after a discharge where return had not previously been expected. It is **not** completed following temporary discharges to hospitals or after therapeutic leaves/home visits.

Resident _____   Numeric Identifier_____

MINIMUM DATA SET (MDS) — *VERSION 2.0*
FOR NURSING HOME RESIDENT ASSESSMENT AND CARE SCREENING
FULL ASSESSMENT FORM
(Status in last 7 days, unless other time frame indicated)

SECTION A. IDENTIFICATION AND BACKGROUND INFORMATION

1.	RESIDENT NAME	
		a. (First) b. (Middle Initial) c. (Last) d. (Jr./Sr.)

2.	ROOM NUMBER	

3.	ASSESSMENT REFERENCE DATE	a. *Last day of MDS observation period* [ ] — [ ] — [ ] Month Day Year b. Original (0) or corrected copy of form (enter number of correction)

4a.	DATE OF REENTRY	Date of reentry from most recent temporary discharge to a hospital in last 90 days (or since last assessment or admission if less than 90 days) [ ] — [ ] — [ ] Month Day Year

5.	MARITAL STATUS	1. Never married 3. Widowed 5. Divorced 2. Married 4. Separated

6.	MEDICAL RECORD NO.	

7.	CURRENT PAYMENT SOURCES FOR N.H. STAY	*(Billing Office to indicate; check all that apply in last 30 days)*
		Medicaid per diem [a.] VA per diem [f.]
		Medicare per diem [b.] Self or family pays for full per diem [g.]
		Medicare ancillary part A [c.] Medicaid resident liability or Medicare co-payment [h.]
		Medicare ancillary part B [d.] Private insurance per diem (including co-payment) [i.]
		CHAMPUS per diem [e.] Other per diem [j.]

8.	REASONS FOR ASSESSMENT *[Note—If this is a discharge or reentry assessment, only a limited subset of MDS items need be completed]*	a. Primary reason for assessment 1. Admission assessment (required by day 14) 2. Annual assessment 3. Significant change in status assessment 4. Significant correction of prior assessment 5. Quarterly review assessment 6. Discharged—return not anticipated 7. Discharged—return anticipated 8. Discharged prior to completing initial assessment 9. Reentry 0. NONE OF ABOVE b. *Special codes for use with supplemental assessment types in Case Mix demonstration states or other states where required* 1. 5 day assessment 2. 30 day assessment 3. 60 day assessment 4. Quarterly assessment using full MDS form 5. Readmission/return assessment 6. Other state required assessment

9.	RESPONSIBILITY/ LEGAL GUARDIAN	*(Check all that apply)*
		Legal guardian [a.] Durable power of attorney/ financial [d.]
		Other legal oversight [b.] Family member responsible [e.]
		Durable power of attorney/health care [c.] Patient responsible for self [f.]
		NONE OF ABOVE [g.]

10.	ADVANCED DIRECTIVES	*(For those items with supporting documentation in the medical record, check all that apply)*
		Living will [a.] Feeding restrictions [f.]
		Do not resuscitate [b.] Medication restrictions [g.]
		Do not hospitalize [c.] Other treatment restrictions [h.]
		Organ donation [d.] NONE OF ABOVE [i.]
		Autopsy request [e.]

SECTION B. COGNITIVE PATTERNS

1.	COMATOSE	*(Persistent vegetative state/no discernible consciousness)* 0. No 1. Yes *(If yes, skip to Section G)*

2.	MEMORY	*(Recall of what was learned or known)*
		 a. Short-term memory OK—seems/appears to recall after 5 minutes
		    0. Memory OK 1. Memory problem **2**
		 b. Long-term memory OK—seems/appears to recall long past
		    0. Memory OK 1. Memory problem **2**

[ ] = When box blank, must enter number or letter.

[a.] = When letter in box, check if condition applies

Code "NA" if information unavailable or unknown.

3.	MEMORY/ RECALL ABILITY	*(Check all that resident was normally able to recall during last 7 days)*
		Current season [a.] That he/she is in a nursing home [d.]
		Location of own room [b.] NONE OF ABOVE are recalled [e.]
		Staff names/faces [c.]

4.	COGNITIVE SKILLS FOR DAILY DECISION-MAKING	*(Made decisions regarding tasks of daily life)* 0. INDEPENDENT—decisions consistent/reasonable 1. MODIFIED INDEPENDENCE—some difficulty in new situations only **2** 2. MODERATELY IMPAIRED—decisions poor; cues/ supervision required **2** 3. SEVERELY IMPAIRED—never/rarely made decisions **2, 5B**

5.	INDICATORS OF DELIRIUM— PERIODIC DISORDERED THINKING/ AWARENESS	*(Code for behavior in the last 7 days.)* [Note: Accurate assessment requires conversations with staff and family who have direct knowledge of resident's behavior over this time.] 0. Behavior not present 1. Behavior present, not of recent onset 2. Behavior present, over last 7 days appears different from resident's usual functioning (e.g., new onset or worsening)
		a. EASILY DISTRACTED—(e.g., difficulty paying attention; gets sidetracked) 2 = **1, 17***
		b. PERIODS OF ALTERED PERCEPTION OR AWARENESS OF SURROUNDINGS—(e.g., moves lips or talks to someone not present; believes he/she is somewhere else; confuses night and day) 2 = **1, 17***
		c. EPISODES OF DISORGANIZED SPEECH—(e.g., speech is incoherent, nonsensical, irrelevant, or rambling from subject to subject; loses train of thought) 2 = **1, 17***
		d. PERIODS OF RESTLESSNESS—(e.g., fidgeting or picking at skin, clothing, napkins, etc.; frequent position changes; repetitive physical movements or calling out) 2 = **1, 17***
		e. PERIODS OF LETHARGY—(e.g., sluggishness; staring into space; difficult to arouse; little body movement) 2 = **1, 17***
		f. MENTAL FUNCTION VARIES OVER THE COURSE OF THE DAY—(e.g., sometimes better, sometimes worse; behaviors sometimes present, sometimes not) 2 = **1, 17***

6.	CHANGE IN COGNITIVE STATUS	Resident's cognitive status, skills, or abilities have changed as compared to status of 90 days ago (or since assessment if less than 90 days) 0. No change 1. Improved 2. Deteriorated **1, 17***

SECTION C. COMMUNICATION/HEARING PATTERNS

1.	HEARING	*(With hearing appliance, if used)* 0. HEARS ADEQUATELY—normal talk, TV, phone 1. MINIMAL DIFFICULTY when not in quiet setting **4** 2. HEARS IN SPECIAL SITUATIONS ONLY—speaker has to adjust tonal quality and speak distinctly **4** 3. HIGHLY IMPAIRED/absence of useful hearing **4**

2.	COMMUNICATION DEVICES/ TECHNIQUES	*(Check all that apply during last 7 days)* Hearing aid, present and used [a.] Hearing aid, present and not used regularly [b.] Other receptive comm. techniques used (e.g., lip reading) [c.] NONE OF ABOVE [d.]

3.	MODES OF EXPRESSION	*(Check all used by resident to make needs known)* Speech [a.] Signs/gestures/sounds [d.] Writing messages to express or clarify needs [b.] Communication board [e.] American sign language or Braille [c.] Other [f.] NONE OF ABOVE [g.]

4.	MAKING SELF UNDERSTOOD	*(Expressing information content—however able)* 0. UNDERSTOOD 1. USUALLY UNDERSTOOD—difficulty finding words or finishing thoughts **4** 2. SOMETIMES UNDERSTOOD—ability is limited to making concrete requests **4** 3. RARELY/NEVER UNDERSTOOD **4**

5.	SPEECH CLARITY	*(Code for speech in the last 7 days)* 0. CLEAR SPEECH—distinct, intelligible words 1. UNCLEAR SPEECH—slurred, mumbled words 2. NO SPEECH—absence of spoken words

6.	ABILITY TO UNDERSTAND OTHERS	*(Understanding verbal information content—however able)* 0. UNDERSTANDS 1. USUALLY UNDERSTANDS—may miss some part/ intent of message **2, 4** 2. SOMETIMES UNDERSTANDS—responds adequately to simple, direct communication **2, 4** 3. RARELY/NEVER UNDERSTANDS **2, 4**

7.	CHANGE IN COMMUNICATION/ HEARING	Resident's ability to express, understand, or hear information has changed as compared to status of 90 days ago (or since last assessment if less than 90 days) 0. No change 1. Improved 2. Deteriorated **17***

Form 1728HF   © 1995 Briggs Corporation, Des Moines, IA 50306   (800) 247-2343   PRINTED IN U.S.A.
 Copyright limited to addition of trigger system.

    MDS 2.0   10/18/94N

Resident _____

SECTION D. VISION PATTERNS		
1.	VISION	*(Ability to see in adequate light and with glasses if used)*
		0. *ADEQUATE*—sees fine detail, including regular print in newspapers/books
		1. *IMPAIRED*—sees large print, but not regular print in newspapers/books [3]
		2. *MODERATELY IMPAIRED*—limited vision; not able to see newspaper headlines, but can identify objects [3]
		3. *HIGHLY IMPAIRED*—object identification in question, but eyes appear to follow objects [3]
		4. *SEVERELY IMPAIRED*—no vision or sees only light, colors, or shapes; eyes do not appear to follow objects
2.	VISUAL LIMITATIONS/ DIFFICULTIES	Side vision problems—decreased peripheral vision (e.g., leaves food on one side of tray, difficulty traveling, bumps into people and objects, misjudges placement of chair when seating self) [3] a.
		Experiences any of following: sees halos or rings around lights; sees flashes of light; sees "curtains" over eyes b.
		NONE OF ABOVE c.
3.	VISUAL APPLIANCES	Glasses; contact lenses; magnifying glass 0. No 1. Yes

SECTION E. MOOD AND BEHAVIOR PATTERNS		
1.	INDICATORS OF DEPRESSION, ANXIETY, SAD MOOD	*(Code for indicators observed in last 30 days, irrespective of the assumed cause)* 0. Indicator not exhibited in last 30 days 1. Indicator of this type exhibited up to five days a week 2. Indicator of this type exhibited daily or almost daily (6, 7 days a week)

VERBAL EXPRESSIONS OF DISTRESS

a. Resident made negative statements—e.g., *"Nothing matters; Would rather be dead; What's the use; Regrets having lived so long; Let me die"* 1 or 2 = **8**

b. Repetitive questions—e.g., *"Where do I go; What do I do?"* 1 or 2 = **8**

c. Repetitive verbalizations—e.g., calling out for help (*"God help me"*) 1 or 2 = **8**

d. Persistent anger with self or others—e.g., easily annoyed, anger at placement in nursing home; anger at care received 1 or 2 = **8**

e. Self deprecation—e.g., *"I am nothing; I am of no use to anyone"* 1 or 2 = **8**

f. Expressions of what appear to be unrealistic fears—e.g., fear of being abandoned, left alone, being with others 1 or 2 = **8**, **17***

g. Recurrent statements that something terrible is about to happen—e.g., believes he or she is about to die, have a heart attack 1 or 2 = **7, 8**

h. Repetitive health complaints—e.g., persistently seeks medical attention, obsessive concern with body functions 1 or 2 = **8**

i. Repetitive anxious complaints/concerns (non-health related) e.g., persistently seeks attention/reassurance regarding schedules, meals, laundry/clothing, relationship issues 1 or 2 = **8**

SLEEP-CYCLE ISSUES

j. Unpleasant mood in morning 1 or 2 = **8**

k. Insomnia/change in usual sleep pattern 1 or 2 = **8**

SAD, APATHETIC, ANXIOUS APPEARANCE

l. Sad, pained, worried facial expressions—e.g., furrowed brows 1 or 2 = **8**

m. Crying, tearfulness 1 or 2 = **8**

n. Repetitive physical movements—e.g., pacing, hand wringing, restlessness, fidgeting, picking 1 or 2 = **8, 17***

LOSS OF INTEREST

o. Withdrawal from activities of interest—e.g., no interest in longstanding activities or being with family/friends 1 or 2 = **7, 8**

p. Reduced social interaction 1 or 2 = **8**

2.	MOOD PERSISTENCE	One or more indicators of depressed, sad or anxious mood were not easily altered by attempts to "cheer up", console, or reassure the resident over last 7 days 0. No mood indicators 1. Indicators present, easily altered **8** 2. Indicators present, not easily altered **8**	
3.	CHANGE IN MOOD	Resident's mood status has changed as compared to status of 90 days ago (or since last assessment if less than 90 days) 0. No change 1. Improved 2. Deteriorated **1, 17***	
4.	BEHAVIORAL SYMPTOMS	*(A) Behavioral symptom frequency in last 7 days* 0. Behavior not exhibited in last 7 days 1. Behavior of this type occurred 1 to 3 days in last 7 days 2. Behavior of this type occurred 4 to 6 days, but less than daily 3. Behavior of this type occurred daily *(B) Behavioral symptom alterability in last 7 days* 0. Behavior not present OR behavior was easily altered 1. Behavior was not easily altered (A) (B)	

a. WANDERING (moved with no rational purpose, seemingly oblivious to needs or safety) A = 1, 2, or 3 = **9, 11**

b. VERBALLY ABUSIVE BEHAVIORAL SYMPTOMS (others were threatened, screamed at, cursed at) A = 1, 2, or 3 = **9**

c. PHYSICALLY ABUSIVE BEHAVIORAL SYMPTOMS (others were hit, shoved, scratched, sexually abused) A = 1, 2, or 3 = **9**

d. SOCIALLY INAPPROPRIATE/DISRUPTIVE BEHAVIORAL SYMPTOMS (made disruptive sounds, noisiness, screaming, self-abusive acts, sexual behavior or disrobing in public, smeared/threw food/feces, hoarding, rummaged through others' belongings) A = 1, 2, or 3 = **9**

e. RESISTS CARE (resisted taking medications/injections, ADL assistance, or eating) A = 1, 2, or 3 = **9**

Numeric Identifier _____

5.	CHANGE IN BEHAVIORAL SYMPTOMS	Resident's behavior status has changed as compared to **status of 90 days ago** (or since last assessment if less than 90 days) 0. No change 1. Improved **9** 2. Deteriorated **1, 17***	

SECTION F. PSYCHOSOCIAL WELL-BEING			
1.	SENSE OF INITIATIVE/ INVOLVE-MENT	At ease interacting with others	a.
		At ease doing planned or structured activities	b.
		At ease doing self-initiated activities	c.
		Establishes own goals **7**	d.
		Pursues involvement in life of facility (e.g., makes/keeps friends; involved in group activities; responds positively to new activities; assists at religious services)	e.
		Accepts invitations into most group activities	f.
		NONE OF ABOVE	g.
2.	UNSETTLED RELATION-SHIPS	Covert/open conflict with or repeated criticism of staff **7**	a.
		Unhappy with roommate **7**	b.
		Unhappy with residents other than roommate **7**	c.
		Openly expresses conflict/anger with family/friends **7**	d.
		Absence of personal contact with family/friends	e.
		Recent loss of close family member/friend	f.
		Does not adjust easily to change in routines	g.
		NONE OF ABOVE	h.
3.	PAST ROLES	Strong identification with past roles and life status **7**	a.
		Expresses sadness/anger/empty feeling over lost roles/status **7**	b.
		Resident perceives that daily routine (customary routine, activities) is very different from prior pattern in the community **7**	c.
		NONE OF ABOVE	d.

SECTION G. PHYSICAL FUNCTIONING AND STRUCTURAL PROBLEMS				
1.	(A) ADL SELF-PERFORMANCE—*(Code for resident's PERFORMANCE OVER ALL SHIFTS during last 7 days*—Not including setup) 0. *INDEPENDENT*—No help or oversight—OR—Help/oversight provided only 1 or 2 times during last 7 days 1. *SUPERVISION*—Oversight, encouragement or cueing provided 3 or more times during last 7 days—OR—Supervision (3 or more times) plus physical assistance provided only 1 or 2 times during last 7 days 2. *LIMITED ASSISTANCE*—Resident highly involved in activity; received physical help in guided maneuvering of limbs or other nonweight bearing assistance 3 or more times—OR—More help provided only 1 or 2 times during last 7 days 3. *EXTENSIVE ASSISTANCE*—While resident performed part of activity, over last 7-day period, help of following type(s) provided 3 or more times: —Weight-bearing support —Full staff performance during part (but not all) of last 7 days 4. *TOTAL DEPENDENCE*—Full staff performance of activity during entire 7 days 8. *ACTIVITY DID NOT OCCUR* during entire 7 days				

			(A) SELF-PERF	(B) SUPPORT
	(B) ADL SUPPORT PROVIDED—*(Code for MOST SUPPORT PROVIDED OVER ALL SHIFTS during last 7 days; code regardless of resident's self-performance classification)* 0. No setup or physical help from staff 1. Setup help only 2. One person physical assist 3. Two+ persons physical assist 8. ADL activity itself did not occur during entire 7 days				
a.	BED MOBILITY	How resident moves to and from lying position, turns side to side, and positions body while in bed A = 1 = **5A**; A = 2, 3, or 4 = **5A, 16**; A = 8 = **16**		
b.	TRANSFER	How resident moves between surfaces—to/from: bed, chair, wheelchair, standing position (EXCLUDE to/from bath/toilet) A = 1, 2, 3, or 4 = **5A**		
c.	WALK IN ROOM	How resident walks between locations in his/her room A = 1, 2, 3, or 4 = **5A**		
d.	WALK IN CORRIDOR	How resident walks in corridor on unit A = 1, 2, 3, or 4 = **5A**		
e.	LOCOMO-TION ON UNIT	How resident moves between locations in his/her room and adjacent corridor on same floor. If in wheelchair, self-sufficiency once in chair A = 1, 2, 3, or 4 = **5A**		
f.	LOCOMO-TION OFF UNIT	How resident moves to and returns from off unit locations (e.g., areas set aside for dining, activities, or treatments). **If facility has only one floor, how resident moves to and from distant areas on the floor.** If in wheelchair, self-sufficiency once in chair A = 1, 2, 3, or 4 = **5A**		
g.	DRESSING	How resident puts on, fastens, and takes off all items of **street** clothing, including donning/removing prosthesis A = 1, 2, 3, or 4 = **5A**		
h.	EATING	How resident eats and drinks (regardless of skill). Includes intake of nourishment by other means (e.g., tube feeding, total parenteral nutrition) A = 1, 2, 3, or 4 = **5A**		
i.	TOILET USE	How resident uses the toilet room (or commode, bedpan, urinal); transfers on/off toilet, cleanses, changes pad, manages ostomy or catheter, adjusts clothes A = 1, 2, 3, or 4 = **5A**		
j.	PERSONAL HYGIENE	How resident maintains personal hygiene, including combing hair, brushing teeth, shaving, applying makeup, washing/drying face, hands, and perineum (EXCLUDE baths and showers) A = 1, 2, 3, or 4 = **5A**		

Resident _____ Numeric Identifier _____

2.	BATHING	How resident takes full-body bath/shower, sponge bath, and transfers in/out of tub/shower (EXCLUDE washing of back and hair). **Code for most dependent** in self-performance and support. A = 1, 2, 3 or 4 = **5A** (A) BATHING SELF-PERFORMANCE codes appear below. 0. Independent—No help provided 1. Supervision—Oversight help only 2. Physical help limited to transfer only 3. Physical help in part of bathing activity 4. Total dependence 8. Activity itself did not occur during entire 7 days (Bathing support codes are as defined in Item 1, code B above)	(A) (B)

3.	TEST FOR BALANCE (See training manual)	*(Code for ability during test in the last 7 days)* 0. Maintained position as required in test 1. Unsteady, but able to rebalance self without physical support 2. Partial physical support during test; or stands (sits) but does not follow directions for test 3. Not able to attempt test without physical help	
		a. Balance while standing	
		b. Balance while sitting—position, trunk control 1, 2, or 3 = **17***	

4.	FUNCTIONAL LIMITATION IN RANGE OF MOTION (see training manual)	*(Code for limitations during last 7 days that interfered with daily functions or placed resident at risk of injury)* **(A) RANGE OF MOTION** **(B) VOLUNTARY MOVEMENT** 0. No limitation 0. No loss 1. Limitation on one side 1. Partial loss 2. Limitation on both sides 2. Full loss	(A) (B)
		a. Neck	
		b. Arm—Including shoulder or elbow	
		c. Hand—Including wrist or fingers	
		d. Leg—Including hip or knee	
		e. Foot—Including ankle or toes	
		f. Other limitation or loss	

5.	MODES OF LOCOMOTION	*(Check all that apply during last 7 days)*	
		Cane/walker/crutch	a.
		Wheeled self	b.
		Other person wheeled	c.
		Wheelchair primary mode of locomotion	d.
		NONE OF ABOVE	e.

6.	MODES OF TRANSFER	*(Check all that apply during last 7 days)*	
		Bedfast all or most of time **16**	a.
		Bed rails used for bed mobility or transfer	b.
		Lifted manually	c.
		Lifted mechanically	d.
		Transfer aid (e.g., slide board, trapeze, cane, walker, brace)	e.
		NONE OF ABOVE	f.

7.	TASK SEGMENTATION	Some or all of ADL activities were broken into subtasks during last 7 days so that resident could perform them 0. No 1. Yes	

8.	ADL FUNCTIONAL REHABILITATION POTENTIAL	Resident believes he/she is capable of increased independence in at least some ADLs **5A**	a.
		Direct care staff believe resident is capable of increased independence in at least some ADLs **5A**	b.
		Resident able to perform tasks/activity but is very slow	c.
		Difference in ADL Self-Performance or ADL Support, comparing mornings to evenings	d.
		NONE OF ABOVE	e.

9.	CHANGE IN ADL FUNCTION	Resident's ADL self-performance status has changed as compared to status of **90 days ago** (or since last assessment if less than 90 days) 0. No change 1. Improved 2. Deteriorated	

SECTION H. CONTINENCE IN LAST 14 DAYS

1.	CONTINENCE SELF-CONTROL CATEGORIES *(Code for resident's PERFORMANCE OVER ALL SHIFTS)* 0. **CONTINENT**—Complete control (includes use of indwelling urinary catheter or ostomy device that does not leak urine or stool) 1. **USUALLY CONTINENT**—BLADDER, incontinent episodes once a week or less; BOWEL, less than weekly 2. **OCCASIONALLY INCONTINENT**—BLADDER, 2 or more times a week but not daily; BOWEL, once a week 3. **FREQUENTLY INCONTINENT**—BLADDER, tended to be incontinent daily, but some control present (e.g., on day shift); BOWEL, 2-3 times a week 4. **INCONTINENT**—Had inadequate control. BLADDER, multiple daily episodes; BOWEL, all (or almost all) of the time		
a.	BOWEL CONTINENCE	Control of bowel movement, with appliance or bowel continence programs, if employed 1, 2, 3 or 4 = **16**	
b.	BLADDER CONTINENCE	Control of urinary bladder function (if dribbles, volume insufficient to soak through underpants), with appliances (e.g., foley) or continence programs, if employed 2, 3 or 4 = **6**	

2.	BOWEL ELIMINATION PATTERN	Bowel elimination pattern regular—at least one movement every three days	a.	Diarrhea	c.
				Fecal impaction **17***	d.
		Constipation **17***	b.	NONE OF ABOVE	e.

3.	APPLIANCES AND PROGRAMS	Any scheduled toileting plan	a.	Did not use toilet room/commode/urinal	f.
		Bladder retraining program	b.	Pads/briefs used **6**	g.
		External (condom) catheter **6**	c.	Enemas/irrigation	h.
		Indwelling catheter **6**	d.	Ostomy present	i.
		Intermittent catheter **6**	e.	NONE OF ABOVE	j.

4.	CHANGE IN URINARY CONTINENCE	Resident's urinary continence has changed as compared to status of **90 days ago** (or since last assessment if less than 90 days) 0. No change 1. Improved 2. Deteriorated	

SECTION I. DISEASE DIAGNOSES

Check only **those diseases that have a relationship to** current ADL status, cognitive status, mood and behavior status, medical treatments, nursing monitoring, or risk of death. (Do not list inactive diagnoses.)

1.	DISEASES	*(If none apply, CHECK the NONE OF ABOVE box)*				
		ENDOCRINE/METABOLIC/NUTRITIONAL		Hemiplegia/Hemiparesis	v.	
				Multiple sclerosis	w.	
		Diabetes mellitus	a.	Paraplegia	x.	
		Hyperthyroidism	b.	Parkinson's disease	y.	
		Hypothyroidism	c.	Quadriplegia	z.	
		HEART/CIRCULATION		Seizure disorder	aa.	
		Arteriosclerotic heart disease (ASHD)	d.	Transient ischemic attack (TIA)	bb.	
		Cardiac dysrhythmias	e.	Traumatic brain injury	cc.	
		Congestive heart failure	f.	**PSYCHIATRIC/MOOD**		
		Deep vein thrombosis	g.	Anxiety disorder	dd.	
		Hypertension	h.	Depression **17***	ee.	
		Hypotension **17***	i.	Manic depression (bipolar disease)	ff.	
		Peripheral vascular disease **16**	j.	Schizophrenia	gg.	
		Other cardiovascular disease	k.	**PULMONARY**		
		MUSCULOSKELETAL		Asthma	hh.	
		Arthritis	l.	Emphysema/COPD	ii.	
		Hip fracture	m.	**SENSORY**		
		Missing limb (e.g., amputation)	n.	Cataracts **3**	jj.	
		Osteoporosis	o.	Diabetic retinopathy	kk.	
		Pathological bone fracture	p.	Glaucoma **3**	ll.	
		NEUROLOGICAL		Macular degeneration	mm.	
		Alzheimer's disease	q.	**OTHER**		
		Aphasia	r.	Allergies	nn.	
		Cerebral palsy	s.	Anemia	oo.	
		Cerebrovascular accident (stroke)	t.	Cancer	pp.	
		Dementia other than Alzheimer's disease	u.	Renal failure	qq.	
				NONE OF ABOVE	rr.	

2.	INFECTIONS	*(If none apply, CHECK the NONE OF ABOVE box)*				
		Antibiotic resistant infection (e.g., Methicillin resistant staph)	a.	Septicemia	g.	
				Sexually transmitted diseases	h.	
		Clostridium difficile (c. diff.)	b.	Tuberculosis	i.	
		Conjunctivitis	c.	Urinary tract infection in last 30 days **14**	j.	
		HIV infection	d.	Viral hepatitis	k.	
		Pneumonia	e.	Wound infection	l.	
		Respiratory infection	f.	NONE OF ABOVE	m.	

3.	OTHER CURRENT OR MORE DETAILED DIAGNOSES AND ICD-9 CODES	Dehydration 276.5 = **14**					
		a. _____			•		
		b. _____			•		
		c. _____			•		
		d. _____			•		
		e. _____			•		

SECTION J. HEALTH CONDITIONS

1.	PROBLEM CONDITIONS	*(Check all problems present in last 7 days unless other time frame is indicated)*				
		INDICATORS OF FLUID STATUS		Dizziness/Vertigo **11, 17***	f.	
		Weight gain or loss of 3 or more pounds within a 7 day period **14**	a.	Edema	g.	
				Fever **14**	h.	
		Inability to lie flat due to shortness of breath	b.	Hallucinations **17***	i.	
		Dehydrated; output exceeds input **14**	c.	Internal bleeding	j.	
				Recurrent lung aspirations in last 90 days **17***	k.	
		Insufficient fluid; did NOT consume all/almost all liquids provided during last 3 days **14**	d.	Shortness of breath	l.	
				Syncope (fainting) **17***	m.	
				Unsteady gait **17***	n.	
		OTHER		Vomiting	o.	
		Delusions	e.	NONE OF ABOVE	p.	

Resident _____   Numeric Identifier _____

2.	**PAIN SYMPTOMS**	*(Code the highest level of pain present in the last 7 days)* **a. FREQUENCY** with which resident complains or shows evidence of pain 0. No pain *(skip to J4)* 1. Pain less than daily 2. Pain daily	**b. INTENSITY** of pain 1. Mild pain 2. Moderate pain 3. Times when pain is horrible or excruciating

3.	**PAIN SITE**	*(If pain present, check all sites that apply in last 7 days)*			
		Back pain	a.	Incisional pain	f.
		Bone pain	b.	Joint pain (other than hip)	g.
		Chest pain while doing usual activities	c.	Soft tissue pain (e.g., lesion, muscle)	h.
		Headache	d.	Stomach pain	i.
		Hip pain	e.	Other	j.

4.	**ACCIDENTS**	*(Check that all apply)*		Hip fracture in **last 180 days 17***	c.
		Fell in **past 30 days** **11, 17***	a.	Other fracture in **last 180 days**	d.
		Fell in **past 31-180 days 11, 17***	b.	*NONE OF ABOVE*	e.

5.	**STABILITY OF CONDITIONS**	Conditions/diseases make resident's cognitive, ADL, mood or behavior patterns unstable—(fluctuating, precarious, or deteriorating)	a.
		Resident experiencing an acute episode or a flare-up of a recurrent or chronic problem	b.
		End-stage disease, 6 or fewer months to live	c.
		NONE OF ABOVE	d.

SECTION K. ORAL/NUTRITIONAL STATUS

1.	**ORAL PROBLEMS**	Chewing problem	a.
		Swallowing problem **17***	b.
		Mouth pain **15**	c.
		NONE OF ABOVE	d.

2.	**HEIGHT AND WEIGHT**	Record *(a.)* height in inches and *(b.)* weight in pounds. Base weight on most recent measure in **last 30 days**; measure weight consistently in accord with standard facility practice— e.g., in a.m. after voiding, before meal, with shoes off, and in nightclothes. **a. HT (in.)** **b. WT (lb.)**

3.	**WEIGHT CHANGE**	**a. Weight loss**—5% or more in **last 30 days**; or 10% or more in **last 180 days** 0. No 1. Yes **12**	
		b. Weight gain—5% or more in **last 30 days**; or 10% or more in **last 180 days** 0. No 1. Yes	

4.	**NUTRITIONAL PROBLEMS**	Complains about the taste of many foods **12**	a.	Leaves 25% or more of food uneaten at most meals **12**	c.
		Regular or repetitive complaints of hunger	b.	*NONE OF ABOVE*	d.

5.	**NUTRITIONAL APPROACHES**	*(Check all that apply in last 7 days)*			
		Parenteral/IV **12, 14**	a.	Dietary supplement between meals	f.
		Feeding tube **13, 14**	b.	Plate guard, stabilized built-up utensil, etc.	g.
		Mechanically altered diet **12**	c.	On a planned weight change program	h.
		Syringe (oral feeding) **12**	d.	*NONE OF ABOVE*	i.
		Therapeutic diet **12**	e.		

6.	**PARENTERAL OR ENTERAL INTAKE**	*(Skip to Section L if neither 5a nor 5b is checked)* **a.** Code the proportion of **total calories** the resident received through parenteral or tube feedings in the **last 7 days** 0. None 3. 51% to 75% 1. 1% to 25% 4. 76% to 100% 2. 26% to 50% **b.** Code the average **fluid intake** per day by IV or tube in **last 7 days** 0. None 3. 1001 to 1500 cc/day 1. 1 to 500 cc/day 4. 1501 to 2000 cc/day 2. 501 to 1000 cc/day 5. 2001 or more cc/day

SECTION L. ORAL/DENTAL STATUS

1.	**ORAL STATUS AND DISEASE PREVENTION**	Debris (soft, easily movable substances) present in mouth prior to going to bed at night **15**	a.
		Has dentures or removable bridge	b.
		Some/all natural teeth lost—does not have or does not use dentures (or partial plates) **15**	c.
		Broken, loose, or carious teeth **15**	d.
		Inflamed gums (gingiva); swollen or bleeding gums; oral abscesses; ulcers or rashes **15**	e.
		Daily cleaning of teeth/dentures or daily mouth care—by resident or staff Not ✓ = **15**	f.
		NONE OF ABOVE	g.

SECTION M. SKIN CONDITION

1.	**ULCERS** (Due to any cause)	*(Record the number of ulcers at each ulcer stage— regardless of cause. If none present at a stage, record "0" (zero). Code all that apply during last 7 days. Code 9 = 9 or more.) [Requires full body exam.]*	**Number at Stage**
		a. Stage 1. A persistent area of skin redness (without a break in the skin) that does not disappear when pressure is relieved.	
		b. Stage 2. A partial thickness loss of skin layers that presents clinically as an abrasion, blister, or shallow crater.	
		c. Stage 3. A full thickness of skin is lost, exposing the subcutaneous tissues—presents as a deep crater with or without undermining adjacent tissue.	
		d. Stage 4. A full thickness of skin and subcutaneous tissue is lost, exposing muscle or bone.	

2.	**TYPE OF ULCER**	*(For each type of ulcer, code for the highest stage in the last 7 days using scale in item M1—i.e., 0=none; stages 1, 2, 3, 4)*	
		a. Pressure ulcer—any lesion caused by pressure resulting in damage of underlying tissue 1 = **16**; 2, 3 or 4 = **12, 16**	
		b. Stasis ulcer—open lesion caused by poor circulation in the lower extremities	

3.	**HISTORY OF RESOLVED ULCERS**	Resident had an ulcer that was resolved or cured in **LAST 90 DAYS** 0. No 1. Yes **16**	

4.	**OTHER SKIN PROBLEMS OR LESIONS PRESENT**	*(Check all that apply during last 7 days)*	
		Abrasions, bruises	a.
		Burns (second or third degree)	b.
		Open lesions other than ulcers, rashes, cuts (e.g., cancer lesions)	c.
		Rashes—e.g., intertrigo, eczema, drug rash, heat rash, herpes zoster	d.
		Skin desensitized to pain or pressure **16**	e.
		Skin tears or cuts (other than surgery)	f.
		Surgical wounds	g.
		NONE OF ABOVE	h.

5.	**SKIN TREATMENTS**	*(Check all that apply during last 7 days)*	
		Pressure relieving device(s) for chair	a.
		Pressure relieving device(s) for bed	b.
		Turning/repositioning program	c.
		Nutrition or hydration intervention to manage skin problems	d.
		Ulcer care	e.
		Surgical wound care	f.
		Application of dressings (with or without topical medications) other than to feet	g.
		Application of ointments/medications (other than to feet)	h.
		Other preventative or protective skin care (other than to feet)	i.
		NONE OF ABOVE	j.

6.	**FOOT PROBLEMS AND CARE**	*(Check all that apply during last 7 days)*	
		Resident has one or more foot problems—e.g., corns, calluses, bunions, hammer toes, overlapping toes, pain, structural problems	a.
		Infection of the foot—e.g., cellulitis, purulent drainage	b.
		Open lesions on the foot	c.
		Nails/calluses trimmed during **last 90 days**	d.
		Received preventative or protective foot care (e.g., used special shoes, inserts, pads, toe separators)	e.
		Application of dressings (with or without topical medications)	f.
		NONE OF ABOVE	g.

SECTION N. ACTIVITY PURSUIT PATTERNS

1.	**TIME AWAKE**	*(Check appropriate time periods over last 7 days)* Resident awake all or most of time (i.e., naps no more than one hour per time period) in the:			
	10B only if BOTH N1a = ✓ and N2 = 0	Morning **10B**	a.	Evening	c.
		Afternoon	b.	*NONE OF ABOVE*	d.

(IF RESIDENT IS COMATOSE, SKIP TO SECTION O)

2.	**AVERAGE TIME INVOLVED IN ACTIVITIES**	*(When awake and not receiving treatments or ADL care)* 0. Most—more than 2/3 of time **10B** 1. Some—from 1/3 to 2/3 of time	2. Little—less than 1/3 of time **10A** 3. None **10A**

3.	**PREFERRED ACTIVITY SETTINGS**	*(Check all settings in which activities are preferred)*			
		Own room	a.		
		Day/activity room	b.	Outside facility	d.
		Inside NH/off unit	c.	*NONE OF ABOVE*	e.

4.	**GENERAL ACTIVITY PREFERENCES** (Adapted to resident's current abilities)	*(Check all PREFERENCES whether or not activity is currently available to resident)*			
				Trips/shopping	g.
		Cards/other games	a.	Walking/wheeling outdoors	h.
		Crafts/arts	b.	Watching TV	i.
		Exercise/sports	c.	Gardening or plants	j.
		Music	d.	Talking or conversing	k.
		Reading/writing	e.	Helping others	l.
		Spiritual/religious activities	f.	*NONE OF ABOVE*	m.

Form 1728HF   © 1995 Briggs Corporation, Des Moines, IA 50306 (800) 247-2343 PRINTED IN U.S.A.
 Copyright limited to addition of trigger system.

MDS 2.0 10/18/94N

Resident _____   Numeric Identifier _____

5.	PREFERS CHANGE IN DAILY ROUTINE	Code for resident preferences in daily routines 0. No change 1. Slight change 2. Major change	
		a. Type of activities in which resident is currently involved 1 or 2 = **10A**	
		b. Extent of resident involvement in activity 1 or 2 = **10A**	

SECTION O. MEDICATIONS

1.	NUMBER OF MEDICATIONS	*(Record the number of different medications used in the last 7 days; enter "0" if none used)*	
2.	NEW MEDICA-TIONS	*(Resident currently receiving medications that were initiated during the last 90 days)* 0. No 1. Yes	
3.	INJECTIONS	*(Record the number of DAYS injections of any type received during the last 7 days; enter "0" if none used)*	
4.	DAYS RECEIVED THE FOLLOWING MEDICATION	*(Record the number of DAYS during last 7 days; enter "0" if not used. Note—enter "1" for long acting meds used less than weekly)* **(NOTE: For 17 to actually be triggered, O4a, b, or c MUST = 1-7 AND at least one additional item marked 17* must be indicated. See sections B, C, E, G, H, I, J, and K.)**	
		a. Antipsychotic 1-7 = **17** d. Hypnotic	
		b. Antianxiety 1-7 = **11, 17** e. Diuretic 1-7 = **14**	
		c. Antidepressant 1-7 = **11, 17**	

SECTION P. SPECIAL TREATMENTS AND PROCEDURES

1.	SPECIAL TREAT-MENTS, PROCE-DURES, AND PROGRAMS	a. SPECIAL CARE—*Check treatments or programs received during the last 14 days*

TREATMENTS				
			Ventilator or respirator	l.
Chemotherapy	a.		**PROGRAMS**	
Dialysis	b.		Alcohol/drug treat-ment program	m.
IV medication	c.		Alzheimer's/dementia special care unit	n.
Intake/output	d.			
Monitoring acute medical condition	e.		Hospice care	o.
Ostomy care	f.		Pediatric unit	p.
Oxygen therapy	g.		Respite care	q.
Radiation	h.		Training in skills required to return to the community (e.g., taking medications, house work, shopping, transportation, ADLs)	r.
Suctioning	i.			
Tracheostomy care	j.			
Transfusions	k.		*NONE OF ABOVE*	s.

b. THERAPIES—*Record the number of days and total minutes each of the following therapies was administered (for at least 15 minutes a day) in the last 7 calendar days (Enter 0 if none or less than 15 min. daily) [Note—count only post admission therapies]* (A) = # of days administered for 15 minutes or more (B) = total # of minutes provided in last 7 days	DAYS (A)	MINUTES (B)
a. Speech-language pathology and audiology services		
b. Occupational therapy		
c. Physical therapy		
d. Respiratory therapy		
e. Psychological therapy (by any licensed mental health professional)		

2.	INTERVEN-TION PROGRAMS FOR MOOD, BEHAVIOR, COGNITIVE LOSS	(Check all interventions or strategies used in **last 7 days**—no matter where received)	
		Special behavior symptom evaluation program	a.
		Evaluation by a licensed mental health specialist in **last 90 days**	b.
		Group therapy	c.
		Resident-specific deliberate changes in the environment to address mood/behavior patterns—e.g., providing bureau in which to rummage	d.
		Reorientation—e.g., cueing	e.
		NONE OF ABOVE	f.

3.	NURSING REHABILI-TATION/RESTOR-ATIVE CARE	Record the NUMBER OF DAYS each of the following rehabilitation or restorative techniques or practices was *provided to the resident for more than or equal to 15 minutes per day in the last 7 days (Enter 0 if none or less than 15 min. daily.)*

a. Range of motion (passive)		f. Walking	
b. Range of motion (active)		g. Dressing or grooming	
c. Splint or brace assistance		h. Eating or swallowing	
TRAINING AND SKILL PRACTICE IN:		i. Amputation/prosthesis care	
d. Bed mobility		j. Communication	
e. Transfer		k. Other	

4.	DEVICES AND RESTRAINTS	*(Use the following codes for last 7 days:)* 0. Not used 1. Used less than daily 2. Used daily	
		Bed rails	
		a. —Full bed rails on all open sides of bed	
		b. —Other types of side rails used (e.g., half rail, one side)	
		c. Trunk restraint 1 = **11, 18**; 2 = **11, 16, 18**	
		d. Limb restraint 1 or 2 = **18**	
		e. Chair prevents rising 1 or 2 = **18**	
5.	HOSPITAL STAY(S)	Record number of times resident was admitted to hospital with an overnight stay in **last 90 days** (or since last assessment if less than 90 days). *(Enter 0 if no hospital admissions)*	
6.	EMERGENCY ROOM (ER) VISIT(S)	Record number of times resident visited ER without an overnight stay in **last 90 days** (or since last assessment if less than 90 days). *(Enter 0 if no ER visits)*	
7.	PHYSICIAN VISITS	In the **LAST 14 DAYS** (or since admission if less than 14 days in facility) how many days has the physician (or authorized assistant or practitioner) examined the resident? *(Enter 0 if none)*	
8.	PHYSICIAN ORDERS	In the **LAST 14 DAYS** (or since admission if less than 14 days in facility) how many days has the physician (or authorized assistant or practitioner) changed the resident's orders? *Do not include order renewals without change. (Enter 0 if none)*	
9.	ABNORMAL LAB VALUES	Has the resident had any abnormal lab values during the last **90 days** (or since admission)? 0. No 1. Yes	

SECTION Q. DISCHARGE POTENTIAL AND OVERALL STATUS

1.	DISCHARGE POTENTIAL	a. Resident expresses/indicates preference to return to the community 0. No 1. Yes	
		b. Resident has a support person who is positive toward discharge 0. No 1. Yes	
		c. Stay projected to be of a short duration—discharge projected **within 90 days** (do not include expected discharge due to death) 0. No 2. Within 31-90 days 1. Within 30 days 3. Discharge status uncertain	
2.	OVERALL CHANGE IN CARE NEEDS	Resident's overall self sufficiency has changed significantly as compared to status of **90 days ago** (or since last assessment if less than 90 days) 0. No change 1. Improved—receives fewer supports, needs less restrictive level of care 2. Deteriorated—receives more support	

SECTION R. ASSESSMENT INFORMATION

1.	PARTICI-PATION IN ASSESSMENT	a. Resident: 0. No 1. Yes	
		b. Family: 0. No 1. Yes 2. No family	
		c. Significant other: 0. No 1. Yes 2. None	

2. SIGNATURES OF PERSONS COMPLETING THE ASSESSMENT:

a. Signature of RN Assessment Coordinator (sign on above line)

b. Date RN Assessment Coordinator signed as complete

	Month		Day		Year

c. Other Signatures	Title	Sections	Date
d.			Date
e.			Date
f.			Date
g.			Date
h.			Date

TRIGGER LEGEND

1 - Delirium	**5B** - ADL-Maintenance	**10A** - Activities (Revise)	**14** - Dehydration/Fluid Maintenance
2 - Cognitive Loss/Dementia	**6B** - Urinary Incontinence and Indwelling Catheter	**10B** - Activities (Review)	**15** - Dental Care
3 - Visual Function	**7** - Psychosocial Well-Being	**11** - Falls	**16** - Pressure Ulcers
4 - Communication	**8** - Mood State	**12** - Nutritional Status	**17** - Psychotropic Drug Use
5A - ADL-Rehabilitation	**9** - Behavioral Symptoms	**13** - Feeding Tubes	**17*** - For this to trigger, O4a, b, or c must = 1-7
			18 - Physical Restraints

MDS 2.0 10/18/94N

SECTION V. RESIDENT ASSESSMENT PROTOCOL SUMMARY   Numeric Identifier_____

Resident's Name:	Medical Record No.:

1. Check if RAP is triggered.

2. For each triggered RAP, use the RAP guidelines to identify areas needing further assessment. Document relevant assessment information regarding the resident's status.

 • Describe:
   —Nature of the condition (may include presence or lack of objective data and subjective complaints).
   —Complications and risk factors that affect your decision to proceed to care planning.
   —Factors that must be considered in developing individualized care plan interventions.
   —Need for referrals/further evaluation by appropriate health professionals.

 • Documentation should support your decision-making regarding whether to proceed with a care plan for a triggered RAP and the type(s) of care plan interventions that are appropriate for a particular resident.

 • Documentation may appear anywhere in the clinical record (e.g., progress notes, consults, flowsheets, etc.).

3. Indicate under the Location of RAP Assessment Documentation column where information related to the RAP assessment can be found.

4. For each triggered RAP, indicate whether a new care plan, care plan revision, or continuation of current care plan is necessary to address the problem(s) identified in your assessment. The Care Planning Decision column must be completed within 7 days of completing the RAI (MDS and RAPs).

A. RAP Problem Area	(a) Check if Triggered	Location and Date of RAP Assessment Documentation	(b) Care Planning Decision—check if addressed in care plan
1. DELIRIUM			
2. COGNITIVE LOSS			
3. VISUAL FUNCTION			
4. COMMUNICATION			
5. ADL FUNCTIONAL/ REHABILITATION POTENTIAL			
6. URINARY INCONTINENCE AND INDWELLING CATHETER			
7. PSYCHOSOCIAL WELL-BEING			
8. MOOD STATE			
9. BEHAVIORAL SYMPTOMS			
10. ACTIVITIES			
11. FALLS			
12. NUTRITIONAL STATUS			
13. FEEDING TUBES			
14. DEHYDRATION/FLUID MAINTENANCE			
15. ORAL/DENTAL CARE			
16. PRESSURE ULCERS			
17. PSYCHOTROPIC DRUG USE			
18. PHYSICAL RESTRAINTS			

B. _____   2. ☐☐ — ☐☐ — ☐☐☐☐
   1. Signature of RN Coordinator for RAP Assessment Process   Month   Day   Year

                                                     4. ☐☐ — ☐☐ — ☐☐☐☐
   3. Signature of Person Completing Care Planning Decision   Month   Day   Year

                                     8 of 8   MDS 2.0 10/18/94N

Appendix E

Other Scales

ABNORMAL INVOLUNTARY MOVEMENT SCALE (AIMS)

Instructions: Complete examination procedure before making ratings. When rating movements, rate highest severity observed and rate movements that occur upon activation one less than those observed spontaneously.

(Put appropriate code in boxes below)

FACIAL AND ORAL MOVEMENTS

1. **Muscles of facial expression**
   e.g., movements of forehead, eyebrows, periorbital area, cheeks; include frowning, blinking, smiling, grimacing.

   0 = None
   1 = Minimal (may be extreme normal)
   2 = Mild
   3 = Moderate
   4 = Severe

2. **Lips and perioral area**
   e.g., puckering, pouting, smacking.

   0 = None
   1 = Minimal (may be extreme normal)
   2 = Mild
   3 = Moderate
   4 = Severe

3. **Jaw**
   e.g., biting, clenching, chewing, mouth opening, lateral movements.

   0 = None
   1 = Minimal (may be extreme normal)
   2 = Mild
   3 = Moderate
   4 = Severe

4. **Tongue**
   Rate only increase in movement both in and out of mouth, **not** inability to sustain movement.

   0 = None
   1 = Minimal (may be extreme normal)
   2 = Mild
   3 = Moderate
   4 = Severe

EXTREMITY MOVEMENTS

5. **Upper (arms, wrists, hands, fingers)**

   Include choreic movements (i.e., rapid, objectively purposeless, irregular, spontaneous) and athetoid movements (i.e., slow, irregular, complex, serpentine). Do **not** include tremor (i.e., repetitive, regular, rhythmic).

   0 = None
   1 = Minimal (may be extreme normal)
   2 = Mild
   3 = Moderate
   4 = Severe

EXTREMITY MOVEMENTS (cont'd)

6. **Lower (legs, knees, ankles, toes)**
   e.g., lateral knee movement, foot tapping, heel dropping, foot squirming, inversion and eversion of foot.

   0 = None
   1 = Minimal (may be extreme normal)
   2 = Mild
   3 = Moderate
   4 = Severe

TRUNK MOVEMENTS

7. **Neck, shoulders, hip**
   e.g., rocking, twisting, squirming, pelvic gyrations.

   0 = None
   1 = Minimal (may be extreme normal)
   2 = Mild
   3 = Moderate
   4 = Severe

GLOBAL JUDGEMENTS

8. **Severity of abnormal movements.**

   0 = None/normal
   1 = Minimal
   2 = Mild
   3 = Moderate
   4 = Severe

9. **Incapacitation due to abnormal movements.**

   0 = None/normal
   1 = Minimal
   2 = Mild
   3 = Moderate
   4 = Severe

10. **Patient's awareness of abnormal movements**
    Rate only patient's report.

    0 = No awareness
    1 = Aware, no distress
    2 = Aware, mild distress
    3 = Aware, moderate distress
    4 = Aware, severe distress

DENTAL STATUS

Any current problems with teeth and/or dentures?   ☐ YES __ NO

Does patient usually wear dentures?   ☐ YES __ NO

Source.   Guy W (ed): *ECDEU Assessment Manual for Psychopharmacology,* Revised Edition. Washington, DC, U.S. Department of Health, Education and Welfare, 1976.

(5/94)

NAME: _____ ID#: _____ DATE: ___/___/___ PERIOD: _____

BEHAVIORAL PATHOLOGY IN ALZHEIMER'S DISEASE (BEHAVE-AD)[1,2]

[BASED UPON INFORMATION OBTAINED FROM CAREGIVER AND/OR OTHER INFORMANTS]

INFORMANT:_____RELATIONSHIP TO PATIENT:_____

PART 1: Symptomatology

(In preceding 2 weeks unless otherwise specified below)

Assessment Interval: _____ weeks

Circle the highest applicable severity rating [0 to 3] for each item. Each category of symptomatology [A to G] is scored independently.

A. Paranoid and Delusional Ideation
(a delusion is a false conviction, not misidentification)

1. <u>"People are stealing things" delusion.</u>

   (0) Not present.
   (1) Delusion that people are hiding objects.
   (2) Delusion that people are coming into the home and hiding or stealing objects.
   (3) Talking and listening to people coming into the home.

2. <u>"One's house is not one's home" delusion.</u>

   (0) Not present.
   (1) Conviction that the place in which one is residing is not one's home
       (e.g., packing to go home, complaints while at home of "take me home").
   (2) Attempt to leave domiciliary to go home.
   (3) Violence in response to attempts to forcibly restrict exit.

3. <u>"Spouse (or other caregiver) is an imposter" delusion.</u>

   (0) Not present.
   (1) Conviction that spouse (or other caregiver) is an imposter.
   (2) Anger towards spouse (or other caregiver) for being an imposter.
   (3) Violence towards spouse (or other caregiver) for being an imposter.

4. <u>Delusion of abandonment (e.g.: to an institution).</u>

   (0) Not present.
   (1) Suspicion of caregiver plotting abandonment or institutionalization (e.g., on the telephone).
   (2) Accusation of a conspiracy to abandon or institutionalize.
   (3) Accusation of impending or immediate desertion or institutionalization.

---

[1] Adapted from Reisberg et al., "Behavioral symptoms in Alzheimer's disease: Phenomenology and treatment," <u>J. Clin. Psychiatry</u>, 1987; 48:5 (Suppl.), 9-15.
[2] © 1986 by Barry Reisberg, M.D. (all rights reserved).

1

BEH - 02

5. <u>Delusion of infidelity</u> (social and/or sexual unfaithfulness).

  (0) Not present.
  (1) Conviction that spouse, children, and/or other caregivers are unfaithful.
  (2) Anger towards spouse, relative, or other caregiver for their infidelity.
  (3) Violence toward spouse, relative, or other caregiver for their infidelity.

6. <u>Suspiciousness/Paranoia other than above.</u>

  (0) Not present.
  (1) Suspiciousness (e.g., hiding objects which they may be unable to locate or a statement such as "I don't trust you").
  (2) Paranoid (i.e., fixed conviction with respect to suspicions and/or anger as a result of suspicions).
  (3) Violence as a result of suspicions.

Unspecified? _____

Describe: _____

_____

_____

_____

_____

7. <u>Delusions (non-paranoid) other than above.</u>

  (0) Not present.
  (1) Delusional.
  (2) Verbal or emotional manifestations as a result of delusions.
  (3) Physical actions or violence as a result of delusions.

Unspecified? _____

Describe: _____

_____

_____

_____

_____

B. Hallucinations

8. Visual hallucinations.

(0) Not present.
(1) Vague, not clearly defined.
(2) Clearly defined hallucinations of objects and persons (e.g., sees other people at the table).
(3) Verbal or physical actions or emotional responses to the hallucinations.

9. Auditory hallucinations.

(0) Not present.
(1) Vague, not clearly defined.
(2) Clearly defined hallucinations of words and phrases.
(3) Verbal or physical actions or emotional responses to the hallucinations.

10. Olfactory hallucinations.

(0) Not present.
(1) Vague, not clearly defined.
(2) Clearly defined hallucinations (e.g., smells a fire or "something burning").
(3) Verbal or physical actions or emotional responses to the hallucinations.

11. Haptic (sense of touch) hallucinations.

(0) Not present.
(1) Vague, not clearly defined.
(2) Clearly defined hallucinations (e.g., "something is crawling on my body").
(3) Verbal or physical actions or emotional responses to the hallucinations.

12. Other hallucinations.

(0) Not present.
(1) Vague, not clearly defined.
(2) Clearly defined hallucinations.
(3) Verbal or physical actions or emotional responses to the hallucinations.

Unspecified? _____

Describe: _____

_____

_____

_____

_____

C. Activity Disturbances.

13. <u>Wandering (e.g., away from home or caregiver)</u>.

(0) Not present.
(1) Somewhat, but not sufficient as to require restraint.
(2) Sufficient as to require restraint.
(3) Verbal or physical actions or emotional responses to attempts to prevent wandering.

14. <u>Purposeless activity (cognitive abulia)</u>.

(0) Not present.
(1) Repetitive, purposeless activity (e.g., opening and closing pocketbook, packing and unpacking clothing, repeatedly putting on and removing clothing, insistent repeating of demands or questions).
(2) Pacing or other purposeless activity sufficient to require restraint.
(3) Abrasions or physical harm resulting from purposeless activity.

15. <u>Inappropriate activity</u>.

(0) Not present.
(1) Inappropriate activities (e.g., storing and hiding objects in inappropriate places, such as throwing clothing in wastebasket or putting empty plates in the oven, inappropriate sexual behavior such as inappropriate exposure).
(2) Present and sufficient to require restraint.
(3) Present and sufficient to require restraint, and accompanied by anger or violence when restraint is used.

Unspecified? _____

Describe: _____

_____

_____

_____

_____

D. Aggressiveness.

16. <u>Verbal Outbursts</u>.

(0) Not present.
(1) Present (including unaccustomed use of foul or abusive language).
(2) Present and accompanied by anger.
(3) Present, accompanied by anger, and clearly directed at other persons.

17. <u>Physical threats and/or violence</u>.

(0) Not present.
(1) Threatening behavior.
(2) Physical violence.
(3) Physical violence accompanied by vehemence.

18. <u>Agitation (other than above)</u>.
   (e.g. non-verbal anger; negativity including refusal to bathe, dress, continue walking, take medications, etc.; hyperventilation).

(0) Not present.
(1) Present.
(2) Present with emotional component.
(3) Present with emotional and physical component.

E. Diurnal Rhythm Disturbances

19. <u>Day/Night disturbance</u>.

(0) Not present.
(2) 50% to 75% of former sleep cycle at night.
(3) Complete disturbance of diurnal rhythm (less than 50% of former sleep cycle at night).

F. Affective Disturbance

20. <u>Tearfulness</u> (or whimpering or other "crying sounds").

   (0) Not present.
   (1) Present.
   (2) Present accompanied by a clear affective component.
   (3) Present and accompanied by affective and physical component
      (e.g., wringing of hands or other gestures).

21. <u>Depressed mood, other</u>.

   (0) Not present.
   (1) Present (e.g., occasional statement "I wish I were dead," or "I'm going to kill myself," or "I feel like
      nothing," without clear affective concomitants).
   (2) Present with clear concomitants (e.g., thoughts of death).
   (3) Present with emotional and physical concomitants (e.g., suicidal gestures).

Unspecified? _____

Describe: _____

_____

_____

_____

_____

G. Anxieties and Phobias

22. <u>Anxiety regarding upcoming events (Godot syndrome).</u>

   (0) Not present.
   (1) Present with repeated queries and/or other activities regarding upcoming appointments and/or
      events (e.g., when are we going?).
   (2) Present and disturbing to caregivers.
   (3) Present and intolerable to caregivers.

23. <u>Other anxieties</u>.
    (e.g., regarding money, the future, being away from home, health, memory, etc.; or generalized anxiety such as thinking everything is "terribly wrong").

   (0) Not present.
   (1) Present.
   (2) Present and disturbing to caregivers.
   (3) Present and intolerable to caregivers.

Unspecified? _____

Describe: _____

_____

_____

_____

_____

_____

24. <u>Fear of being left alone</u>.

   (0) Not present.
   (1) Present with vocalized fear of being alone.
   (2) Vocalized and sufficient to require specific action on the part of caregiver.
   (3) Vocalized and sufficient to require patient to be accompanied at all times (e.g., patient must see the caregiver at all times).

25. <u>Other phobias</u>.
    (e.g. fear of crowds, travel, darkness, people/strangers, bathing, etc.)

   (0) Not present.
   (1) Present
   (2) Present and of sufficient magnitude to require specific action by caregiver.
   (3) Present and sufficient to prevent patient activities.

Unspecified? _____

Describe: _____

_____

_____

_____

_____

TOTAL **SEVERITY** SCORE: _____

BEH-08

PART 2: Global Rating

Circle one choice. Are the symptoms which have been noted of sufficient magnitude as to be:

(0) Not at all troubling to the caregiver or dangerous to the patient.
(1) Mildly troubling to the caregiver or dangerous to the patient.
(2) Moderately troubling to the caregiver or dangerous to the patient.
(3) Severely troubling to the caregiver or dangerous to the patient.

Symptom most troubling to caregiver

"With respect to the above symptoms, which is the biggest problem for you and/or other caregivers?"
(More than one symptom can be listed, but please give numerical order.)

_____

_____

_____

_____

_____

_____

Clinician: _____ Date: _____/_____/_____

Comments: _____

_____

_____

BRIEF PSYCHIATRIC RATING SCALE (BPRS)

Please enter the score for the term which best describes the patient's condition.

0 = not assessed, **1** = not present, **2** = very mild, **3** = mild, **4** = moderate, **5** = moderately severe, **6** = severe, **7** = extremely severe

1. SOMATIC CONCERN
Degree of concern over present bodily health. Rate the degree to which physical health is perceived as a problem by the patient, whether complaints have a realistic basis or not.

SCORE ☐

2. ANXIETY
Worry, fear, or over-concern for present or future. Rate solely on the basis of verbal report of patient's own subjective experiences. Do not infer anxiety from physical signs or from neurotic defense mechanisms.

SCORE ☐

3. EMOTIONAL WITHDRAWAL
Deficiency in relating to the interviewer and to the interviewer situation. Rate only the degree to which the patient gives the impression of failing to be in emotional contact with other people in the interview situation.

SCORE ☐

4. CONCEPTUAL DISORGANIZATION
Degree to which the thought processes are confused, disconnected, or disorganized. Rate on the basis of integration of the verbal products of the patient; do not rate on the basis of patient's subjective impression of his own level of functioning.

SCORE ☐

5. GUILT FEELINGS
Over-concern or remorse for past behavior. Rate on the basis of the patient's subjective experiences of guilt as evidenced by verbal report with appropriate affect; do not infer guilt feelings from depression, anxiety or neurotic defenses.

SCORE ☐

6. TENSION
Physical and motor manifestations of tension "nervousness", and heightened activation level. Tension should be rated solely on the basis of physical signs and motor behavior and not on the basis of subjective experiences of tension reported by the patient.

SCORE ☐

7. MANNERISMS AND POSTURING
Unusual and unnatural motor behavior, the type of motor behavior which causes certain mental patients to stand out in a crowd of normal people. Rate only abnormality of movements; do not rate simple heightened motor activity here.

SCORE ☐

8. GRANDIOSITY
Exaggerated self-opinion, conviction of unusual ability or powers. Rate only on the basis of patient's statements about himself or self-in-relation-to-others, not on the basis of his demeanor in the interview situation.

SCORE ☐

9. DEPRESSIVE MOOD
Despondency in mood, sadness. Rate only degree of despondency; do not rate on the basis of inferences concerning depression based upon general retardation and somatic complaints.

SCORE ☐

10. HOSTILITY
Animosity, contempt, belligerence, disdain for other people outside the interview situation. Rate solely on the basis of the verbal report of feelings and actions of the patient toward others; do not infer hostility from neurotic defenses, anxiety, nor somatic complaints. *(Rate attitude toward interviewer under "uncooperativeness")*.

SCORE ☐

11. SUSPICIOUSNESS
Belief *(delusional or otherwise)* that others have now, or have had in the past, malicious or discriminatory intent toward the patient. On the basis of verbal report, rate only those suspicions which are currently held whether they concern past or present circumstances.

SCORE ☐

12. HALLUCINATORY BEHAVIOR
Perceptions without normal external stimulus correspondence. Rate only those experiences which are reported to have occurred within the last week and which are described as distinctly different from the thought and imagery processes of normal people.

SCORE ☐

13. MOTOR RETARDATION
Reduction in energy level evidenced in slowed movements. Rate on the basis of observed behavior of the patient only; do not rate on the basis of patient's subjective impression of own energy level.

SCORE ☐

14. UNCOOPERATIVENESS
Evidence of resistance, unfriendliness, resentment and lack of readiness to cooperate with the interviewer. Rate only on the basis of the patient's attitude and responses to the interviewer and the interview situation; do not rate on basis of reported resentment or uncooperativeness outside the interview situation.

SCORE ☐

15. UNUSUAL THOUGHT CONTENT
Unusual, odd, strange or bizarre thought content. Rate here the degree of unusualness, not the degree of disorganization of thought processes.

SCORE ☐

16. BLUNTED AFFECT
Reduced emotional tone, apparent lack of normal feeling or involvement.

SCORE ☐

17. EXCITEMENT
Heightened emotional tone, agitation, increased reactivity.

SCORE ☐

18. DISORIENTATION
Confusion or lack of proper association for person, place or time.

SCORE ☐

Source. Overall JE, Gorham DR: "The Brief Psychiatric Rating Scale." *Psychological Reports* 10:799–812, 1962.

Cornell Scale
for Depression in Dementia

NAME _____ AGE _____ SEX _____ DATE _____

WING _____ ROOM _____ PHYSICIAN _____ ASSESSOR _____

Ratings should be based on symptoms and signs occurring during the week before interview. No score should be given if symptoms result from physical disability or illness.

SCORING SYSTEM
a = Unable to evaluate   0 = Absent   1 = Mild to intermittent   2 = Severe

a 0 1 2

A. MOOD-RELATED SIGNS

1. Anxiety: anxious expression, rumination, worrying
2. Sadness: sad expression, sad voice, tearfulness
3. Lack of reaction to present events
4. Irritability: annoyed, short tempered

a 0 1 2

B. BEHAVIORAL DISTURBANCE

5. Agitation: restlessness, hand wringing, hair pulling
6. Retardation: slow movements, slow speech, slow reactions
7. Multiple physical complaints (score 0 if gastrointestinal symptoms only)
8. Loss of interest: less involved in usual activities (score only if change occurred acutely, i.e., in less than one month)

a 0 1 2

C. PHYSICAL SIGNS

9. Appetite loss: eating less than usual
10. Weight loss (score 2 if greater than 5 pounds in one month)
11. Lack of energy: fatigues easily, unable to sustain activities

a 0 1 2

D. CYCLIC FUNCTIONS

12. Diurnal variation of mood: symptoms worse in the morning
13. Difficulty falling asleep: later than usual for this individual
14. Multiple awakening during sleep
15. Early morning awakening: earlier than usual for this individual

a 0 1 2

E. IDEATIONAL DISTURBANCE

16. Suicidal: feels life is not worth living
17. Poor self-esteem: self-blame, self-depreciation, feelings of failure
18. Pessimism: anticipation of the worst
19. Mood congruent delusions: delusions of poverty, illness or loss

SCORE _____	**Score greater than 12 = Probable Depression**

Notes/Current Medications: _____
_____

Source.   Alexopoulos GS, Abrams RC, Young RC, et al: "Cornell Scale for Depression in Dementia." *Biological Psychiatry* 23:271–284, 1988. Used with permission.

Instructions for use:
(Cornell Dementia Depression Assessment Tool)

1. The same CNA (certified nursing assistant) should conduct the interview each time to assure consistency in response.

2. The assessment should be based on the patient's normal weekly routine.

3. If uncertain of answers, questioning other caregivers may further define the answer.

4. Answer all questions by placing a check in the column under the appropriately numbered answer. (a = unable to evaluate, 0 = absent, 1 = mild to intermittent, 2 = severe).

5. Add the total score for all numbers checked for each question.

6. Place the total score in the "SCORE" box and record any subjective observation notes in the "NOTES/CURRENT MEDICATIONS" section.

7. Scores totaling twelve (12) points or more indicate probable depression.

Geriatric Depression Scale

1. Are you basically satisfied with your life ?	yes / no
2. Have you dropped many of your activities and interests ?	yes / no
3. Do you feel that your life is empty ?	yes / no
4. Do you often get bored ?	yes / no
5. Are you hopeful about the future ?	yes / no
6. Are you bothered by thoughts you can't get out of your head ?	yes / no
7. Are you in good spirits most of the time ?	yes / no
8. Are you afraid that something bad is going to happen to you ?	yes / no
9. Do you feel happy most of the time ?	yes / no
10. Do you often feel helpless ?	yes / no
11. Do you often get restless and fidgety ?	yes / no
12. Do you prefer to stay at home, rather than going out and doing new things ?	yes / no
13. Do you frequently worry about the future ?	yes / no
14. Do you feel you have more problems with memory than most ?	yes / no
15. Do you think it is wonderful to be alive now ?	yes / no
16. Do you often feel downhearted and blue ?	yes / no
17. Do you feel pretty worthless the way you are now ?	yes / no
18. Do you worry a lot about the past ?	yes / no
19. Do you find life very exciting ?	yes / no
20. Is it hard for you to get started on new projects ?	yes / no
21. Do you feel full of energy ?	yes / no
22. Do you feel that your situation is hopeless ?	yes / no
23. Do you think that most people are better off than you are ?	yes / no
24. Do you frequently get upset over little things ?	yes / no
25. Do you frequently feel like crying ?	yes / no
26. Do you have trouble concentrating ?	yes / no
27. Do you enjoy getting up in the morning ?	yes / no
28. Do you prefer to avoid social gatherings ?	yes / no
29. Is it easy for you to make decisions ?	yes / no
30. Is your mind as clear as it used to be ?	yes / no

Copyright 1981, J. Yesavage, T. Brink

This is the scoring for the scale : One point for each of these answers.
Cutoff : normal— 0-9 ; mild depressives— 10-19 ; severe depressives— 20-30.

1. no	6. yes	11. yes	16. yes	21. no	26. yes
2. yes	7. no	12. yes	17. yes	22. yes	27. no
3. yes	8. yes	13. yes	18. yes	23. yes	28. yes
4. yes	9. no	14. yes	19. no	24. yes	29. no
5. no	10. yes	15. no	20. yes	25. yes	30. no

The Geriatric Depression Scale questionnaire.

Yesavage JA, Brink TL, Rose TL, Lum O, Huang V, Adey MB, Leirer VO : Development and validation of a geriatric depression screening scale : A preliminary report. J. Psychiatric Research 17 : 37–49, 1983.

Hamilton Depression Rating Scale

Patient's Name _____   Date of First Report _____

Diagnosis _____   Date of This Report _____

Current Therapy _____

Instructions   _For each item check the box next to the response that best characterizes the patient._

Depressed Mood	0 ☐ 1 ☐ 2 ☐ 3 ☐ 4 ☐	Absent. These feeling states indicated only on questioning. These feeling states spontaneously reported verbally. Communicates feeling states nonverbally – ie, through facial expression, posture, voice, and tendency to weep. Patient reports _virtually only_ these feeling states in his spontaneous verbal and non-verbal communication.	_Feelings of sadness, hopelessness, helplessness, worthlessness._
Feelings of Guilt	0 ☐ 1 ☐ 2 ☐ 3 ☐ 4 ☐	Absent. Self-reproach, feels he has let people down. Ideas of guilt or rumination over past errors or sinful deeds. Present illness is a punishment. Delusions of guilt. Hears accusatory or denunciatory voices and/or experiences threatening visual hallucinations.	
Suicide	0 ☐ 1 ☐ 2 ☐ 3 ☐ 4 ☐	Absent. Feels life is not worth living. Wishes he were dead or any thoughts of possible death to self. Suicide ideas or gestures. Attempts at suicide _(only serious attempt rates 4)._	
Insomnia Early	0 ☐ 1 ☐ 2 ☐	No difficulty. Complains of occasional difficulty falling asleep – ie, more than ½ hour. Complains of nightly difficulty falling asleep.	
Insomnia Middle	0 ☐ 1 ☐ 2 ☐	No difficulty. Patient complains of being restless and disturbed during the night. Waking during the night – any getting out of bed rates 2 _(except for purposes of voiding)._	
Insomnia Late	0 ☐ 1 ☐ 2 ☐	No difficulty. Waking in early hours of the morning but goes back to sleep. Unable to fall asleep again if gets out of bed.	
Work and Activities	0 ☐ 1 ☐ 2 ☐ 3 ☐ 4 ☐	No difficulty. Thoughts and feelings of incapacity, fatigue or weakness related to activities; work or hobbies. Loss of interest in activity; hobbies or work – either directly reported by patient, or indirect in listlessness, indecision or vacillation _(feels he has to push self to work or activities)._ Decrease in actual time spent in activities or decrease in productivity. In hospital, rate 3 if patient does not spend at least three hours a day in activities _(hospital job or hobbies)_, exclusive of ward chores. Stopped working because of present illness. In hospital, rate 4 if patient engages in no activities except ward chores, or if patient fails to perform ward chores unassisted.	
Retardation	0 ☐ 1 ☐ 2 ☐ 3 ☐ 4 ☐	Normal speech and thought. Slight retardation at interview. Obvious retardation at interview. Interview difficult. Complete stupor.	_Slowness of thought and speech; impaired ability to concentrate; decreased motor activity._
Agitation	0 ☐ 1 ☐ 2 ☐	None. "Playing with" hands, hair, etc. Hand-wringing, nail-biting, hair-pulling, biting of lips.	
Anxiety Psychic	0 ☐ 1 ☐ 2 ☐ 3 ☐ 4 ☐	No difficulty. Subjective tension and irritability. Worrying about minor matters. Apprehensive attitude apparent in face or speech. Fears expressed without questioning.	

Source.   Hamilton M: "A Rating Scale for Depression." _Journal of Neurology, Neurosurgery and Psychiatry_ 23:56–62, 1960.

Hamilton Depression Rating Scale

Anxiety Somatic	0 ☐ 1 ☐ 2 ☐ 3 ☐ 4 ☐	Absent. Mild. Moderate. Severe. Incapacitating.	*Physiological concomitants of anxiety, such as:* *Gastrointestinal – dry mouth, wind, indigestion, diarrhea, cramps, belching.* *Cardiovascular – palpitations, headaches.* *Respiratory – hyperventilation, sighing.* *Urinary frequency.* *Sweating.*
Somatic **Symptoms** **Gastrointestinal**	0 ☐ 1 ☐ 2 ☐	None. Loss of appetite but eating without staff encouragement. Heavy feelings in abdomen. Difficulty eating without staff urging. Requests or requires laxatives or medication for bowels or medication for GI symptoms.	
Somatic **Symptoms** **General**	0 ☐ 1 ☐ 2 ☐	None. Heaviness in limbs, back or head. Backaches, headache, muscle aches. Loss of energy or fatigability. Any clear-cut symptom rates 2.	
Genital **Symptoms**	0 ☐ 1 ☐ 2 ☐	Absent. Mild. Severe.	*Symptoms such as:* *Loss of libido.* *Menstrual disturbances.*
Hypochondriasis	0 ☐ 1 ☐ 2 ☐ 3 ☐ 4 ☐	Not present. Self-absorption (bodily). Preoccupation with health. Frequent complaints, requests for help, etc. Hypochondriacal delusions.	
Loss of **Weight** (Answer only A or B)	 0 ☐ 1 ☐ 2 ☐ 0 ☐ 1 ☐ 2 ☐	**A. When rating by history:** No weight loss. Probable weight loss associated with present illness. Definite (according to patient) weight loss. **B. On weekly ratings by ward psychiatrist, when actual weight changes are measured:** Less than 1 lb weight loss in week. Greater than 1 lb weight loss in week. Greater than 2 lb weight loss in week.	
Insight	0 ☐ 1 ☐ 2 ☐	Acknowledges being depressed and ill. Acknowledges illness but attributes cause to bad food, climate, overwork, virus, need for rest, etc. Denies being ill at all.	
Diurnal **Variation**	 ☐ ☐ ☐ 1 ☐ 2 ☐	**Note whether symptoms are worse in the morning or evening.** No variation. Worse in AM. Worse in PM. **When present, rate the variation.** Mild. Severe.	
Depersonalization **and** **Derealization**	0 ☐ 1 ☐ 2 ☐ 3 ☐ 4 ☐	Absent. Mild. Moderate. Severe. Incapacitating.	*Such as:* *Feelings of unreality.* *Nihilistic ideas.*
Paranoid **Symptoms**	0 ☐ 1 ☐ 2 ☐ 3 ☐	None. Suspicious. Ideas of reference. Delusions of reference and persecution.	
Obsessional **and Compulsive** **Symptoms**	0 ☐ 1 ☐ 2 ☐	Absent. Mild. Severe.	

Total Score

Instrumental Activities of Daily Living (IADL) Scale

Subject's Name _____ Rated by _____ Date _____

Agency:_____ Informant _____

Circle one statement in each category A–H that applies to subject.

A. Ability to use telephone

1. Operates telephone on own initiative—looks up and dials numbers, etc.
2. Dials a few well-known numbers.
3. Answers telephone but does not dial.
4. Does not use telephone at all.

B. Shopping

1. Takes care of all shopping needs independently.
2. Shops independently for small purchases.
3. Needs to be accompanied on any shopping trip.
4. Completely unable to shop.

C. Food preparation

1. Plans, prepares, and serves adequate meals independently.
2. Prepares adequate meals if supplied with ingredients.
3. Heats and serves prepared meals, or prepares meals but does not maintain adequate diet.
4. Needs to have meals prepared and served.

D. Housekeeping

1. Maintains house alone or with occasional assistance (e.g., "heavy work—domestic help").
2. Performs light daily tasks such as dishwashing, bedmaking.
3. Performs light daily tasks but cannot maintain acceptable level of cleanliness.
4. Needs help with all home maintenance tasks.
5. Does not participate in any housekeeping tasks.

E. Laundry

1. Does personal laundry completely.
2. Launders small items—rinses socks, stockings, etc.
3. All laundry must be done by others.

Source. Lawton MP, Brody EM: "Assessment of Older People: Self-Maintaining and Instrumental Activities of Daily Living." *Gerontologist* 9:179–186, 1969.

IADL *(continued)*

F. **Mode of transportation**

1. Travels independently on public transportation or drives own car.
2. Arranges own travel via taxi, but does not otherwise use public transportation.
3. Travels on public transportation when assisted or accompanied by another.
4. Travel limited to taxi or automobile with assistance of another.
5. Does not travel at all.

G. **Responsibility for own medications**

1. Is responsible for taking medication in correct dosages at correct time.
2. Takes responsibility if medication is prepared in advance in separate dosages.
3. Is not capable of dispensing own medication.

H. **Ability to handle finances**

1. Manages financial matters independently (budgets, writes checks, pays rent, bills, goes to bank) collects and keeps track of income.
2. Manages day-to-day purchases, but needs help with banking, major purchases, etc.
3. Incapable of handling money.

MiniMental LLC

THE ANNOTATED MINI MENTAL STATE EXAMINATION (AMMSE)

NAME OF SUBJECT _____ Age _____

NAME OF EXAMINER _____ Years of School Completed ____

Approach the patient with respect and encouragement.
Ask: Do you have any trouble with your memory? ☐ Yes ☐ No
May I ask you some questions about your memory? ☐ Yes ☐ No

Date of Examination _____

SCORE	ITEM

5 ( )   TIME ORIENTATION

Ask:

What is the year_____(1), season_____(1),

month of the year_____(1), date_____(1),

day of the week_____(1) ?

5 ( )   PLACE ORIENTATION

Ask:

Where are we now? What is the state_____(1), city_____(1),

part of the city_____(1), building_____(1),

floor of the building_____(1)?

3 ( )   REGISTRATION OF THREE WORDS

Say: Listen carefully. I am going to say three words. You say them back after I stop.

Ready? Here they are... PONY (wait 1 second), QUARTER (wait 1 second), ORANGE (wait one

second). What were those words?

_____(1)

_____(1)

_____(1)

Give 1 point for each correct answer, then repeat them until the patient learns all three.

5 ( )   SERIAL 7 s AS A TEST OF ATTENTION AND CALCULATION

Ask: Subtract 7 from 100 and continue to subtract 7 from each subsequent remainder

until I tell you to stop. What is 100 take away 7 ?_____(1)

Say:

Keep Going. _____(1),_____(1),

_____(1)_____(1),

3 ( )   RECALL OF THREE WORDS

Ask:

What were those three words I asked you to remember?

Give one point for each correct answer_____(1),

_____(1), _____(1),

For more
information or
additional copies
of this exam,
call (617)587-4215

2 ( )   NAMING

Ask:

What is this? (show pencil)_____(1). What is this? (show watch)_____(1).

© 1975, 1998 MiniMental, LLC

O V E R

Source. Folstein MF, Folstein SE, McHugh PR: "'Mini-Mental State': A Practical Method for Grading the Cognitive State of Patients for the Clinician." *Journal of Psychiatric Research* 12:189–198, 1975. The copyright in the Mini Mental State Examination is wholly owned by the MiniMental LLC, a Massachusetts limited liability company. For information about how to obtain permission to use or reproduce the Mini Mental State Examination, please contact John Gonsalves Jr., Administrator of the MiniMental LLC, at 31 St. James Avenue, Suite I, Boston, MA 02116, 617-587-4215. Copyright © 1975, 1998 MiniMental LLC.

MiniMental LLC

1 ( )   **REPETITION**

Say:

Now I am going to ask you to repeat what I say. Ready? No ifs, ands, or buts.

Now you say that. _____ (1)

3 ( )   **COMPREHENSION**

Say:

Listen carefully because I am going to ask you to do something:

Take this paper in your left hand (1), fold it in half (1), and put it on the floor. (1)

1 ( )   **READING**

Say:

Please read the following and do what it says, but do not say it aloud.   (1)

Close your eyes

1 ( )   **WRITING**

Say:

Please write a sentence. If patient does not respond, say: Write about the weather. (1)

_____

_____

1 ( )   **DRAWING**

Say: Please copy this design.

TOTAL SCORE _____   Assess level of consciousness along a continuum

Alert	Drowsy	Stupor	Coma

	YES	NO
Cooperative:	☐	☐
Depressed:	☐	☐
Anxious:	☐	☐
Poor Vision:	☐	☐
Poor Hearing:	☐	☐
Native Language:		

	YES	NO
Deterioration from previous level of functioning:	☐	☐
Family History of Dementia:	☐	☐
Head Trauma:	☐	☐
Stroke:	☐	☐
Alcohol Abuse:	☐	☐
Thyroid Disease:	☐	☐

FUNCTION BY PROXY

Please record date when patient was last able to perform the following tasks.
Ask caregiver if patient independently handles:

	YES	NO	DATE
Money/Bills:	☐	☐	____
Medication:	☐	☐	____
Transportation:	☐	☐	____
Telephone:	☐	☐	____

Appendix F

Suggested Reading

Abrams WB, Beers MH, Berkow R: The Merck Manual of Geriatrics, 2nd Edition. Whitehouse Station, NJ, Merck, 1995

American Psychiatric Association: Practice guideline for the treatment of patients with Alzheimer's disease and other dementias of late life. Am J Psychiatry 154 (suppl 5), 1997

Billig N: Growing Older and Wiser. New York, Lexington Books, 1993

Birkett DP: Psychiatry in the Nursing Home: Assessment, Evaluation, and Intervention. New York, Haworth, 1991

Birkett DP: The Psychiatry of Stroke. Washington, DC, American Psychiatric Press, 1996

Blazer DG: Depression in Late Life, 2nd Edition. St. Louis, MO, Mosby–Year Book, 1993

Burns T, Mortimer JA, Merchak P: Cognitive performance test: a new approach to functional assessment in Alzheimer's disease. Journal of Geriatric Psychiatry and Neurology 7:46–54, 1994

Busse EW, Blazer DG (eds): Textbook of Geriatric Psychiatry, 3rd Edition. Washington, DC, American Psychiatric Press, 2000

Cassel CK, Cohen HJ, Larson EB, et al (eds): Geriatric Medicine, 3rd Edition. New York, Springer, 1997

Coffey CE, Cummings JL (eds): Textbook of Geriatric Neuropsychiatry. Washington, DC, American Psychiatric Press, 1994

Copeland JRM, Abou-Saleh MT, Blazer DG (eds): Principles and Practice of Geriatric Psychiatry. West Sussex, England, Wiley, 1994

Duthie EH, Katz PR: Practice of Geriatrics, 3rd Edition. Philadelphia, PA, WB Saunders, 1998

Greene JA: Creative Aging, 1995 [Available from James A. Greene, M.D., 9040 Executive Park Drive, Suite 107, Knoxville, TN 37923-4630]

Jarvik LF, Winograd CH: Treatments for the Alzheimer Patient. New York, Springer, 1988

Kapp MB: Medicolegal issues, in Psychiatric Care in the Nursing Home. Edited by Reichman WE, Katz PR. New York, Oxford University Press, 1996

Lawlor BA (ed): Behavioral Complications in Alzheimer's Disease. Washington, DC, American Psychiatric Press, 1995

Mace NL, Rabins PV: The 36-Hour Day, Revised Edition. Baltimore, MD, Johns Hopkins University Press, 1991

The OBRA '87 enforcement rule: implications for attending physicians and medical directors. American Medical Directors Association, Columbia, MD, 1995

Ouslander JG, Osterweil D, Morley J: Medical Care in the Nursing Home, 2nd Edition. New York, McGraw-Hill, 1997

Pattee JJ, Otteson OJ: Medical Direction in the Nursing Home: Principles and Concepts for Physician Administrators. Minneapolis, MN, North Ridge Press, 1991

Reichman WE, Katz PR: Psychiatric Care in the Nursing Home. New York, Oxford University Press, 1996

Sadavoy J, Lazarus LW, Jarvik LF, et al (eds): Comprehensive Review of Geriatric Psychiatry, 2nd Edition. Washington, DC, American Psychiatric Press, 1996

Salzman C: Clinical Geriatric Psychopharmacology, 3rd Edition. Baltimore, MD, Williams & Wilkins, 1998

Siegal AP, Jackson JM, Moak G, et al: Geriatric Psychiatry: Practice Management Handbook. Bethesda, MD, American Association for Geriatric Psychiatry, 1997

Smith DA: Geriatric Psychopathology: Behavioral Intervention as First Line Treatment. Providence, RI, Manisses Communications Group, 1995

Williams ME: The American Geriatrics Society's Complete Guide to Aging and Health. New York, Harmony Books, 1995

Index

*Page numbers printed in **boldface** type refer to tables or figures.*

Manual of nursing home
practice for psychiatrists